Clinician's Guide
to MIND OVER MOOD

Clinician's Guide
to
MIND OVER MOOD

CHRISTINE A. PADESKY, PH.D.

with DENNIS GREENBERGER, PH.D.

THE GUILFORD PRESS
New York   London

Printed in the United States of America

This book is printed on acid-free paper.

Last digit is print number: 9 8 7 6 5 4 3 2 1

Library of Congress Cataloging-in-Publication Data is available
from the Publisher.

ISBN 0-89862-821-0

Designed and formatted by
KP Company
Brooklyn, NY

Preface

Many photographers travel with only a wide-angle and a telephoto lens. A wide-angle lens allows for a full-horizon view of any scene. A telephoto lens allows the photographer to either bring a distant point closer or view something nearby in great detail. As therapists, we use both wide-angle and telephoto perspectives with every client we see.

This week we may see people who are depressed, anxious, struggling with relationship problems, recovering from serious trauma, confronting substance abuse, or adjusting to another type of change. To be effective, we must be able to understand, conceptualize, and know how to skillfully apply treatment plans for the broad spectrum of human problems in increasingly brief periods of time.

We need the perspective of a wide-angle lens to consider a range of options, and the power of a telephoto lens to bring treatment goals into proximate focus. This book shows how the client treatment manual *Mind Over Mood* can assist in accomplishing these therapy tasks. Chapters in this therapist guide offer suggestions for integrating the treatment manual into therapy, outline strategies for helping clients set therapy goals, and provide directions for using the treatment manual with a variety of client problems in a variety of treatment settings.

Most therapists are familiar with the cognitive therapy approach. Cognitive therapy is the fastest growing form of psychotherapy. Its rapid growth has been attributed to its clarity, proven effectiveness, and philosophical "fit" with the information-processing Zeitgeist of the last two decades. Further, there has been a growing demand by consumers and third-party payors for brief yet effective therapies. Cognitive therapy successfully meets these demands. *Mind Over Mood* makes these psychotherapy advances available to more clients. This therapist guide teaches how to use *Mind Over Mood* and individualize it for each client for maximum therapy effectiveness.

Acknowledgments

When we finished writing *Mind Over Mood: A Cognitive Therapy Treatment Manual* for *Clients*, our editor asked us to write an additional book for clinicians describing how to use the client treatment manual. Since I had been teaching cognitive therapy training courses for therapists for more than a decade, I agreed to write most of this book which shows how to integrate the client manual with cognitive therapy treatment protocols. Dennis Greenberger agreed to write chapters on group therapy and inpatient therapy, two areas in which he has extensive clinical expertise.

My own excitement regarding this book was matched by that of our editor, Kitty Moore. During this past year, Kitty has been supportive, constructively critical, and creative in her contributions. I deeply appreciate her humor, patience, and good counsel throughout this project. Many times, her encouraging voice at the other end of the phone gave me the necessary energy boost to complete one more round of revisions and additions.

The material in this book was derived from workshops I've taught since 1978. Throughout this time, Aaron T. Beck has been a generous mentor and friend, offering me many high profile workshop opportunities early in my career so that I could follow my heart and become a near full-time teacher of cognitive therapy. Many of the researchers and clinicians cited and referenced in this clinician's guide are personal friends as well as colleagues. Without the collective research and theoretical and clinical talent of this group, cognitive therapy would not be as effective and this book could not have been written.

vii

Due to tight time deadlines, no one other than our editor, Dennis, and myself read the entire manuscript prior to its final stages. Instead, portions of particular chapters were given to colleagues with special expertise in those areas. Paul Salkovskis reviewed portions of an early draft of the anxiety chapter. Jan Scott read many of the chapters and offered useful suggestions and references for the depression and inpatient chapters. Nancy Waite-O'Brien shared her ideas on how *Mind Over Mood* could help solve problems faced in substance abuse treatment. Patrice Yasuda offered feedback and references regarding use of cognitive therapy with people of various cultures. Kathleen Mooney, Marlyn Osborn, Karen Simon, and Gail Simpson read the early chapters of this guide for clarity and completeness. Participants in Camp Cognitive Therapy III reviewed the brief therapy chapter. Since these colleagues only read portions of early drafts out of context, any errors or deficiencies remaining in this text are my own responsibility.

In order to write this book in the six-month time frame requested, I needed to stop most of my other professional activities. Special thanks are due to Kathleen Mooney and Karen Simon, psychologists at the Center for Cognitive Therapy in Newport Beach, who stepped in and accepted additional administrative and clinical responsibilities so I could spend days on end at the computer.

Thanks are also due to my friends and family who tolerated my social absences, fatigue, and detailed book discussions over the past year. Two of these friends loaned and eventually gave me a notebook computer so I could literally write everywhere. Others agreed to cook late night dinners. Still others offered good humor and encouraging conversation when my spirits flagged. For these and many other forms of support I especially thank Anne, Brian, Barbara, Barbra, Bill, Bob, Brenda, Diane, Dick, Donella, Gillian, Helen, Jan, Kathleen, Kevin, Marc, Matt, Rose, Rosanne, Scott, Sharon, Skip, Stacey, Sue, Tim, and my parents.

And finally, I thank you, the reader. Anticipating your needs and questions kept me up at night and also helped me maintain enthusiasm for this project. I hope this book helps you share our vision for how *Mind Over Mood* can enhance your clinical work.

CHRISTINE A. PADESKY, June 1995

My contributions to this book were influenced by many people. Art Freeman deserves special recognition for sparking my interest in cognitive therapy. Judy Beck and Aaron T. Beck later fueled that spark and provided ongoing encouragement for this project.

In addition to her formidable editing skills, Kitty Moore guided and counseled me throughout the writing of my chapters. Her contributions cannot be overestimated.

Diedre Greenberger's love and support helped me see this project through to completion. Elysa and Alanna's spirit and energy provide focus, perspective, and meaning to my life.

DENNIS GREENBERGER, June 1995

Contents

1

How to Use MIND OVER MOOD in Therapy

A new client, Joan, arrives for an intake appointment. In this first meeting, you learn that Joan is depressed, has a five-year history of cocaine abuse, recently became unemployed, and has concerns about her teenage son's truancy from school. Joan is still covered by the insurance plan from her previous job. Her mental health benefits allow eight outpatient therapy sessions and do not allow family therapy. Joan seems motivated to make a change in her life, and you think you could help her more if you weren't limited to eight sessions.

Peter, age 36, began therapy six months ago when his father died. With a 20-year history of generalized anxiety disorder, Peter was skeptical that therapy could help. However, he now sees you as someone who can help him find his way in life. Peter has adopted a dependent style in therapy.

He presents you with a new problem each week and asks you for guidance. When you ask Peter what he has learned in previous discussions that might help solve his current problems, he replies, "I don't know. When I get anxious I can't remember what we've said."

How often do you face these types of scenarios? Many clients, like Joan, need more therapy than we can provide. Others, like Peter, need to independently apply what is discussed in therapy. Joan, Peter, and their therapists would benefit from the use of a client treatment manual such as *Mind Over Mood: A Cognitive Therapy Treatment Manual for Clients.*

A client treatment manual provides a structure for therapeutic intervention beyond the therapy hour. Joan's therapist could use therapy sessions to construct plans to solve the crises and problems in Joan's life and help Joan enroll in a drug treatment program. The therapist could assign chapters in *Mind Over Mood* to be read between therapy appointments to help Joan learn skills to lessen her depression and cope with the thoughts and feelings maintaining her cocaine use. The client manual might provide enough support so that Joan's last two or three appointments could be spaced several weeks apart without jeopardizing Joan's progress. Joan could also use the client manual after therapy has ended to guide continued improvement.

A client treatment manual also helps summarize and organize learning so that clients can remember and use what has been discussed in therapy. Peter's therapist could recommend *Mind Over Mood* as a tool for fostering independent problem solving. The exercises in the manual would help Peter learn skills to help manage his own anxiety. For Peter, the client manual would provide a bridge between reliance on his therapist and dependence on himself. Undoubtedly, Peter's feelings and thoughts about becoming independent would emerge as he began to use the manual. The feelings and thoughts could be discussed in therapy sessions and also explored by Peter on the worksheets in *Mind Over Mood.*

Many therapists have never used a client treatment manual as part of therapy. Figure 1.1 provides a decision tree to help you decide if the manual might be helpful. This chapter provides specific suggestions to help you integrate *Mind Over Mood* into therapy. Subsequent chapters in this book specify treatment protocols for using *Mind Over Mood* with a range of client problems to provide focused

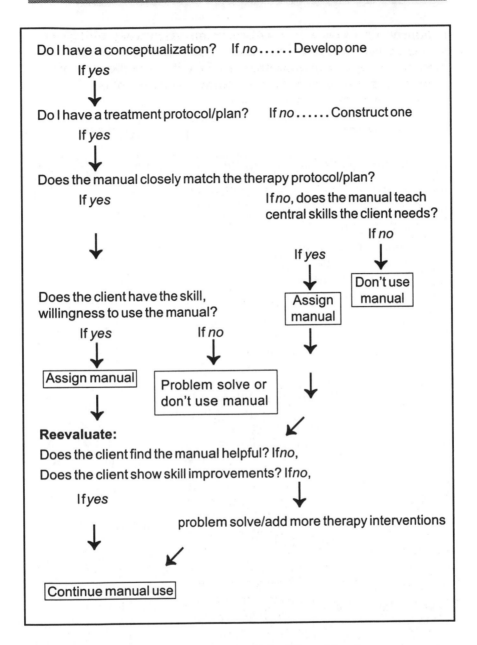

FIGURE 1.1. Decision tree for use of *Mind Over Mood.*

treatment for a variety of client problems in a variety of treatment settings. Since *Mind Over Mood* is a cognitive therapy (CT) treatment manual, we begin with a discussion of the critical components of cognitive therapy and how to use a client treatment manual in CT.

A QUICK GUIDE TO COGNITIVE THERAPY

A complete description of cognitive therapy includes cognitive theory (e.g., Beck et al., 1990; Beck, Rush, Shaw, & Emery, 1979), cognitive models for case conceptualization (see Beck et al., 1990; Persons, 1989), and specific treatment protocols for different client problems. Cognitive therapy texts that provide full descriptions of the therapy are cited throughout this book and can be consulted for elaboration of the theory and treatment approaches.

Cognitive therapists assess thoughts, moods, behaviors, biology, and environment in understanding the origin of client problems. These five areas of life are interconnected, each part influencing the others. Although cognitive therapists may intervene in any or all of the five areas to help a client, cognitive therapy places particular emphasis on identifying and evaluating thoughts and on behavioral change.

The focus on thoughts does not mean that cognitive therapists believe that thoughts cause all problems. However, thoughts play a powerful role in maintaining dysfunctional moods and behaviors regardless of their origins. For example, a woman may become depressed following a great personal loss in combination with a genetic predisposition toward depression. Even if her depression is conceptualized as resulting from environmental and biological stressors, a cognitive focus would be an important part of the treatment. Once depressed, her thoughts become characteristically negative, as described by Beck (1967).

Each emotional state, regardless of origin, is accompanied by characteristic patterns of thinking. Anxiety is accompanied by thoughts of danger and vulnerability; anger by thoughts of violation and unfairness. Therapeutic change is hampered if these thoughts are not identified and evaluated. For example, the course of treatment for the depressed woman might include establishing supportive relationships in her time of loss. She might refuse to make these contacts because of characteristic thinking patterns that occur in depression: "It won't help" (hopelessness), "I'm no fun to be around" (self-criticism), and "I don't enjoy myself anyway" (global negativity).

Cognitive therapists teach clients to identify, evaluate, and change dysfunctional thinking patterns so that therapeutic changes in mood and behavior can occur. These changes often help clients change their environment (e.g., "If I have worth, maybe I deserve more nurturing relationships") and may be accompanied by biological shifts. Three levels of thoughts are addressed in cognitive therapy: automatic thoughts, underlying assumptions, and schemas (the less technical term "core beliefs" is used in *Mind Over Mood*).

Automatic thoughts are the moment-to-moment, unplanned thoughts (words, images, and memories) that flow through our minds throughout the day. Underlying assumptions are cross-situational beliefs or rules that guide our lives; they include "should" statements ("A woman should always think of her children first") and conditional "if . . . then" beliefs ("If people get to know me, they will reject me"). Underlying assumptions guide behavior and expectations, although often they are not articulated consciously.

Schemas have been described as screens or filters that process and code stimuli (Beck et al., 1979). In this clinician's guide, the word *schema* is used to describe absolutistic core beliefs about the self, others and the world. Schemas are absolute ("I am strong") and dichotomous ("I am strong," " I am weak"). As discussed in Chapter 7 of this guide, schemas are central in the treatment of clients with personality disorders and other lifelong problems.

The three levels of thought are interconnected. Schemas ("I'm unlovable") give birth to underlying assumptions ("If people meet me, they won't like me"); together they determine what types of automatic thoughts occur ("I won't have any fun at the party" is more likely to accompany an unlovability schema than "I'll go to the party and make some friends"). Many cognitive therapy texts label only two levels of thought, automatic thoughts and schemas. We believe three levels are helpful because therapists can differentially choose therapy methods based on the type of thought to be evaluated. Automatic thoughts are best evaluated on Thought Records (*Mind Over Mood*, Chapters 4–7), underlying assumptions are usually tested with behavioral experiments (*Mind Over Mood*, Chapter 8) and change in schemas is effected by learning to rate experiences on a continuum and to use a variety of core belief logs (*Mind Over Mood*, Chapter 9).

Understanding the interplay between levels of thought and moods, behavior, physical functions, and environment is central to cognitive theory and practice. Two fundamental clinical processes underlie the therapy itself: a collaborative therapy relationship and guided discovery. Since these two factors are critical to the successful use of *Mind Over Mood*, suggestions for implementing them are described here.

Establishing a Collaborative Therapy Relationship

A positive therapist–client relationship is a critically important foundation for successful therapy. Clients are most likely to honestly and openly discuss problems in a relationship that seems safe and trustworthy. The best cognitive therapists are warm, empathic, and genuine with their clients, qualities basic to any good therapeutic relationship. These qualities are demonstrated in the therapist's straightforward curiosity about the client's experiences, thoughts, and feelings and by the efforts the therapist makes to devise a brief and effective therapy plan to help the client improve quickly. To fit with this type of therapy relationship, a treatment manual should be introduced to the client as a caring assist to client progress, not as a therapist convenience.

Cognitive therapy adds "collaborative" to the list of qualities important to the therapy relationship. Collaboration requires an active stance on the part of both therapist and client to work together as a team. Since many clients enter therapy expecting to play a more passive role ("Fix me"), the therapist often needs to socialize the client to expectations for mutual collaboration.

A collaborative therapist conveys to clients that they have important information that must be shared to solve problems. The therapist knows general strategies and treatment models, and the client holds all the information about his or her unique experiences and is the only one who can describe thoughts and moods. The client's experience dictates how general principles will be applied to help current problems. Collaboration also allows the client to give feedback to the therapist and ask questions to learn as much as possible to make informed choices and decisions. In cognitive therapy, the therapist agrees to respect and encourage collaborative exchanges.

A warm therapy relationship without visible progress in solving presenting problems can actually make a client feel worse over time. *Mind Over Mood* helps establish a collaborative therapy relationship that promotes client progress in three ways. First, the manual encourages client independence from the therapist in learning therapeutic approaches to solving problems. The more a client learns to solve problems independently, the greater the chances he or she will take the steps necessary for life improvement. Second, the worksheets in the manual actively enlist the client's efforts to apply what is learned in therapy to everyday life experiences. The worksheets highlight the client's observations and insight. Worksheets are reviewed in therapy as a visible record of learning and participation. Third, the worksheets provide immediate feedback to client and therapist about whether the client understands the skills taught in therapy and whether the skills are helpful in correcting target problems.

If actual or perceived violations in trust, confidence, interpersonal comfort, or respect disrupt the therapy relationship, client progress may suffer. Therefore, the therapist should regularly ask the client for feedback about the therapy relationship and procedures. If clients are asked for feedback about therapy progress and the therapy relationship in each session, they become more comfortable raising concerns as they arise. Any disruptions in collaboration should be discussed and mutually resolved as soon as possible.

As an example, Roy said that he thought his therapist was trying to hurry him out the door at the end of each session. Notice how the therapist respectfully collaborated with Roy to solve the problem.

T: We have only five minutes left today, so let me get some feedback from you on how the therapy is going for you and any reactions you might have to our relationship.

R: Well, it's going pretty OK.

T: You say that with some hesitation. Is there something that could be better for you?

R: Yes. It's this endpoint every week. I don't like the idea that you watch the clock. It's like you want to hurry me out of here.

T: What exactly do I do that gives you that impression?

R: Well, you always tell me when there are a few minutes left. And I always leave between ten and five minutes before the hour is up. I thought therapy was a whole hour long.

T: And so you figure that means I am hurrying you out faster than usual.

R: Yes.

T: And how does that feel to you?

R: I feel like I'm unimportant to you.

T: Does that make you feel sad? or angry? or something else?

R: A little angry. I want to have my full amount of time.

T: I'm very glad you're bringing this up today. Do you have more to say about what this means to you, or would you like to hear what it means to me?

R: I would like to know how you feel.

T: First, I'm not aware of feelings that I want to hurry you out of here. However, its always possible I am feeling pressured to hurry sometimes. Although I don't think that has to do with you personally, I will pay attention to my feelings to see if those feelings are there. If so, I'll try to figure out with you what prompts them and how we can work together to keep a good relationship.

R: But you seem so aware of the time.

T: Does it seem that way to you the entire session or just at the end?

R: Not in the beginning or middle. Just at the end when you get me to leave early.

T: This is where I have done a poor job of communicating to you, Roy. You see, I try to end all my appointments ten minutes before the hour. I use the time after you leave and before my next appointment to make notes on what we talked about and to write myself reminders of what topics I think it is important for us to discuss in the next session. Before we meet, I read those notes and try to get myself ready to continue our work together. So, while we only meet for *50* minutes, I spend about an hour on each session.

R: I wondered how you remembered so much about me.

T: Just as I ask you to write things down between sessions, I need to do that too. I should have explained this to you clearly at the first session so you knew to expect only a 50-minute meeting. I'm sorry.

R: Well, I feel better knowing you do this with everyone.

T: I wonder if the way I tell you there is only five minutes left also makes it harder for you in some way.

R: Yes. I know why you do it. But it surprises me sometimes because some weeks the time goes so quickly.

T: What would it be like for you if I didn't say, "Five minutes left"?

R: (*Pause*) It would be worse for me if the end of the session came and I wasn't expecting it.

T: I do let you know so we can cover whatever else is important to you to discuss. But maybe there's a better way for me to signal you.

R: I have a setting on my watch to make it beep at a certain time every hour. Maybe I could set it to go off at 5:45, and then we'd know.

T: That's a great idea. Would you be willing to do that?

R: Yes. And then I'd feel a little more in control of our time.

T: Let's try that next week. Let's also both think more about this discussion to see if there is more to say. I'm going to make a note that you feel better when you are in control of the time. We may want to look more at this issue of feeling in control because it might relate to some of your relationship problems we've been discussing.

R: OK.

T: Before you leave, how are you feeling right now about our relationship and what we've just discussed?

R: Better. I was nervous bringing this up, but I'm glad I did.

T: I am, too. Please bring up any other concerns you have so we can have a chance to work them out together.

R: OK. I will.

In this therapy excerpt the therapist truly collaborates with Roy in exploring his concerns. She asks him to describe his thoughts and feelings about session endings and also discusses her own thoughts and feelings. Rather than seeing the issue as all internal to Roy, she takes responsibility for her inadequate communication to him about session time. Once the situation is mutually understood, Roy and the therapist discuss mutually agreeable solutions. If Roy did not suggest his wristwatch, the therapist might suggest placing a clock in the therapy room so that they could both keep track of the time. Or they might agree that she will continue to note when the session is almost over. Collaboration implies mutual problem solving rather than one-sided decision-making. For example, the therapist would not accept a request from Roy that sessions last until he feels ready to end.

Although almost all clients who used earlier versions of *Mind*

Over Mood responded positively, use of a client treatment manual may occasionally create friction in the therapy relationship. Therapists who follow the guidelines for using the client manual described in this clinician's guide will rarely encounter difficulties in its use. However, a few clients may have negative reactions to the idea of using a manual. Chapter 7 of this guide describes several negative client reactions to a client manual and explicit therapeutic strategies for responding to them.

Guiding Client Discovery

A second cornerstone of cognitive therapy is guided discovery. Imagine a depressed client who says, "I'm a complete failure." If you say to this client, "Wait a minute. You are successful in work, you have three nice children, and your life is generally good. How is that a failure?" the client is likely to respond, "You don't understand . . . " or "Yes, but . . ." Offering an alternative viewpoint to a distressed client is rarely helpful if done directly.

To help clients avoid global judgments of experience and construct more balanced views, cognitive therapists use guided discovery (see Beck, Rush, Shaw, & Emery, 1979). Rather than directly pointing out information that contradicts a depressed client's negative beliefs, a cognitive therapist asks a series of questions to help the client discover alternative meanings. The following therapist–client dialogue illustrates this process.

C: I'm a complete failure.

T: How long have you been feeling this way?

C: Just a few months. But I see now it has always been true.

T: What makes you think you're a failure?

C: I haven't accomplished anything of lasting value.

T: I see. No wonder you're discouraged. I'm a bit confused about something, though.

C: What's that?

T: Do you think any of the work you've done over the past ten years has lasting value—for you or for someone else?

C: Well, I don't know . . . I suppose some of the people our agency helps have benefitted.

T: Has your work contributed in any way to these benefits?

C: Yes. I have helped a number of people over the years. Others I've not been able to help.

T: So you've helped some people, not others.

C: Yes.

T: How about at home? Have you contributed anything to your family of value to you or to them?

C: My kids seem happy with me. I think I've been a good parent. But I can see lots of ways I could be a better parent.

T: If you want, we can talk about that. But first, I'm wondering how the people you've helped at work and the good things you've done as a parent fit with the idea that you haven't accomplished anything of value.

C: They don't, really. I guess I have done some things that are good. But when I get down, all I can see is the fly in the ointment.

T: OK. That's helpful to know. Let's talk about the fly in the ointment that's bothering you right now. And let's also keep in mind your observation that you've had some accomplishments in your life, even if they are hard to remember when you're depressed.

As this therapist–client dialogue shows, a few minutes of questioning can help a client develop an alternative perspective that the client finds credible because it is based on information provided by the client, not the therapist. Practice will help you master the art of using questions to guide discovery.

HELPFUL HINTS

☞

Guided Discovery (Padesky, 1993a)

Guided discovery generally consists of

1. a series of questions to uncover relevant information outside the client's current awareness

2. accurate listening and reflection by the therapist

3. a summary of information discovered

4. a synthesizing question that asks the client to apply the new information discussed to his or her original belief

Mind Over Mood is written in the style of guided discovery. Each chapter asks questions to guide clients' discovery of key principles. Worksheets help clients summarize the information discovered and apply learning principles to their own beliefs and life problems. Therapists can pattern their own questioning in therapy sessions on the types of questions provided in the client manual. For example, Chapter 5 of *Mind Over Mood* lists questions that are useful in uncovering key automatic thoughts. Chapter 6 lists questions that can uncover information that contradicts a maladaptive belief.

Good questioning strategies are only a part of guided discovery. It is also important that both therapist and client use an experimental approach to evaluating beliefs, behaviors, moods, and plans for change. *Mind Over Mood* facilitates this aspect of guided discovery by encouraging clients to test beliefs, experiment with new behaviors, consider alternate interpretations for events, and conduct experiments to evaluate the worthiness of action plans for change. The four clients described in *Mind Over Mood* illustrate these aspects of guided discovery by expressing skepticism (Ben in the opening pages of Chapter 1), struggling with data that are hard to accept (Marissa in Chapter 6), and conducting experiments to try to change both emotional reactions and behavior (Linda and Vic in Chapter 8). Thus, *Mind Over Mood* supports the commitment to curiosity and exploration that the cognitive therapist establishes in the therapy session.

Even deciding with a client whether or not to use a treatment manual can be part of guided discovery in therapy. Therapist and client can discuss the pros and cons of a manual and use it experimentally for a few weeks to see how it helps or hinders therapy progress. In addition, therapist and client can experiment with different uses for the manual, as described later in this chapter. For example, therapist and client could work together on manual worksheets in two sessions and the client could work alone on worksheets between two subsequent sessions. Then client and therapist could begin to evaluate whether and how much therapist guidance is necessary to maximize client learning from the manual.

The following sections show you how to introduce *Mind Over Mood* to your clients, integrate the manual with your in-session therapy work, increase client compliance in using the manual, and troubleshoot common difficulties that may arise. Our recommendations show how these tasks can be accomplished following the two basic principles of cognitive therapy, collaboration and guided discovery.

INTRODUCING *MIND OVER MOOD*
TO YOUR CLIENT

How many psychotherapy books are sitting on your shelf that you have not read? Most therapists have several such books if not a bookshelf full. Presumably you bought these books because you thought they would be helpful or interesting. What determines which books you read and use?

The first goal in introducing a client to *Mind Over Mood* is to increase the likelihood that the manual will be read and used. It is important to allow time in the therapy session to describe or show the book to your client, give a rationale for its use, discuss your mutual expectations for how it might be helpful in therapy, and present clear instructions on how you would like your client to use the book in subsequent weeks. One way to introduce *Mind Over Mood* follows. Note how the therapist uses collaboration and guided discovery to facilitate her client's interest in using the manual.

T: You've been very specific today in describing your anxiety to me. If I've heard you correctly, you feel anxious all the time.

C: Yes, I can hardly stand it.

T: Most people who are anxious want to get over it as quickly as possible. Do you feel that way?

C: Oh, yes.

T: One of the things I've learned in helping people overcome anxiety is that we get results faster if we take some time early in therapy to learn as much as possible about the anxiety before we try to get rid of it. For example, if you just took a tranquilizer or avoided the situations in which you feel anxious you might feel calmer, but we still wouldn't know what was behind your anxiety. Once you stopped the medication or couldn't avoid any longer, you'd be back in the same place. Do you understand what I mean?

C: You're saying I need to go through the anxiety to learn about it?

T: Yes. Does that make sense to you?

C: I think I understand, but I don't like it.

T: Being anxious isn't fun. So we better make sure we learn something from your anxiety to help you.

C: I'm not sure what I'll learn.

T: In the beginning, it would help if you could make some observations about your anxiety. When does it increase or decrease? What goes through your mind when you are anxious? What do you feel physically? This information can help us figure out together what your anxiety is all about and how to best help you.

C: OK. But I'm not exactly sure how to do that.

T: There is a lot *to* learn in the beginning of therapy. I'd like to recommend a book to you that can help you learn about your anxiety in between our appointments. Do you think a written reminder of what we've talked about and some written instructions about how to observe your anxiety would help you?

C: Sure.

T: As you see, the book is called *Mind Over Mood*. It's called that because we're going to discover how your thoughts are connected to your anxiety and whether or not changes in your thinking can reduce your anxiety. As you'll learn in the first chapter, anxiety is connected to thoughts, behaviors, physical functions, and the events in someone's life. We'll need your observations to find out if this is true for you.

C: Should I read the whole book?

T: This book isn't meant to be read in one week. If you like the book, we'll use it to help us throughout therapy. Read just the first chapter before our next appointment, and see if you can fill out Worksheet 1.1 on understanding your problems by following the instructions in the chapter. Then bring the book to therapy next week so that we can look at the worksheet together. If you have any problems with it, I'll help you next time.

C: OK.

T: If you want to do more, you could also read Chapter 11, which is about anxiety. Some of the information in Chapter 11 reviews what we talked about today and some of it will be new to you. If you do read Chapter 11, fill out the anxiety questionnaire on page 178 so that we know how anxious you are now, and we'll aim to help you become less anxious in a few weeks. Do you think you'll have time to read Chapter 11, or do you just want to read Chapter 1?

C: I might have time.

T: You could see how Chapter 1 goes and then decide if you want to read the first part of Chapter 11. Why don't you circle on the table of contents what you've agreed to do this week so you don't forget.

(Client circles Chapter 1, writes "If I have time" next to Chapter 11.)

T: Is there anything that might get in the way of reading the first chapter this week?

C: No. It doesn't look too hard.

T: If you have difficulty, I'll help you next time. But I think you'll find this interesting. I'm certainly curious to learn more about what things are connected to your anxiety. So bring the book back next week, even if you don't complete everything. OK?

C: OK.

The therapist in this example does not hurry the discussion of *Mind Over Mood*. She introduces the manual during the session at a point when the client is expressing a need that might be helped by the manual ("I'm not exactly sure how to do that"). She also gives a rationale for using a treatment manual (it will "help you learn" between appointments, provide a written reminder of what has been discussed in therapy, instruct you how to observe anxiety) and clear instructions on what portions of the manual to complete in the following week.

Further, the therapist collaborates with the client, asking with each request if the client is willing to comply and also giving the client a choice about how much reading to do. The therapist asks about roadblocks that might interfere with the reading and offers to help if the client is not able to complete the assignment. These communications imply that the manual is intended to help the client, not be a burdensome task. Finally, the therapist signals that the manual will be an integral part of the next session ("bring the book back next week") and expresses her own interest and curiosity in discovering what the client will learn.

As this example illustrates, a few minutes of discussion linking *Mind Over Mood* to the therapy goals and learning process can weave the manual into the fabric of the therapy contract. Clients are more likely to actively use the manual if therapists encourage its use outside therapy and its review inside therapy sessions. Clients with whom we have used the manual bring it and any other therapy notebooks or journals they keep to each session, and we discuss or review the writings and observations pertinent to that week's learning.

Before using *Mind Over Mood* with clients, therapists are advised to familiarize themselves with its contents. The more thoroughly you know the manual, the easier it will be to tailor assignments to a particular client. Further, particular chapters or worksheets can be used in therapy sessions, as described in the next section. Weaving the treatment manual into therapy encourages client use of the manual outside sessions and provides a bridge toward independent practice of therapy skills learned. Finally, the client manual provides many "Helpful Hints" boxes and several "Troubleshooting Guides" that therapists can use to navigate "stuck" points in therapy sessions. Reading *Mind Over Mood* carefully may help improve the quality of therapy you provide by suggesting change strategies and paths for client discovery that are new to you.

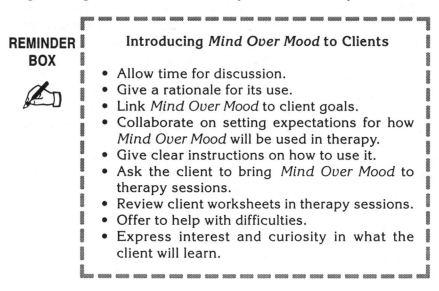

REMINDER BOX

Introducing *Mind Over Mood* to Clients

- Allow time for discussion.
- Give a rationale for its use.
- Link *Mind Over Mood* to client goals.
- Collaborate on setting expectations for how *Mind Over Mood* will be used in therapy.
- Give clear instructions on how to use it.
- Ask the client to bring *Mind Over Mood* to therapy sessions.
- Review client worksheets in therapy sessions.
- Offer to help with difficulties.
- Express interest and curiosity in what the client will learn.

ENHANCING THERAPY WITH *MIND OVER MOOD*

Once you have made the choice to integrate *Mind Over Mood* with therapy, you can use the treatment manual in a variety of ways. Three different uses are described here: (1) as a template for treatment, (2) as an adjunct to treatment, and (3) to pinpoint specific skills development.

Using *Mind Over Mood* as a Template for Treatment

For many clients, *Mind Over Mood* provides a useful step-by-step treatment plan with little modification or additional information needed. Clients who are depressed, experience generalized anxiety disorder, or meet the criteria for some personality disorders (e.g., avoidant, dependent, obsessive–compulsive, and borderline personality disorders) may benefit from a cognitive therapy treatment plan that focuses almost exclusively on teaching the skills described in the client manual. (Chapters 4 through 7 of the clinician's guide describe in detail how to use *Mind Over Mood* in treating such clients). Therapists who lead skills development therapy groups (Chapter 9) or who offer brief therapy to clients struggling with mood-related problems (Chapters 4, 5, and 8) can also use *Mind Over Mood* as a ready-made treatment program.

If *Mind Over Mood* is used as the core of therapy, the therapist should make sure the client is interested in the manual and is able to use it. Most clients welcome use of a treatment manual because they can set their own learning pace—and a manual can reduce the cost of therapy. Therapist and client should discuss how much help the client would like and how frequently sessions should be scheduled. Meeting weekly the first two or three weeks is often ideal because the therapist needs to assess the client's problems and determine whether a treatment manual is appropriate to the therapy. Also, the therapist can use the initial therapy sessions to help the client set reasonable therapy goals (following the guidelines in Chapter 3 of the clinician's guide) and to review the client's response to the initial chapters of the treatment manual.

If a client responds with interest and successfully completes the first few chapters of *Mind Over Mood*, it may be possible to meet less frequently in subsequent weeks. This therapy course is illustrated in the following case example.

———

Pam, struggling with depression, an alcoholic husband, and a variety of family crises, came to therapy requesting help to "cope better." She and the therapist decided after the first meeting that she would benefit from cognitive therapy for depression, Al-Anon, support in getting her husband to treatment, and the development of assertion skills so that she could say no to family members who made unreasonable demands of her. Pam had limited financial resources and her health insurance plan covered eight therapy sessions. When offered *Mind Over Mood* as a core part of therapy, she eagerly agreed to give it a try.

After the first session, Pam read and completed Chapter 1 (Understanding Your Problems) and Chapter 2 (It's the Thought That Counts). The therapist reviewed her worksheets in the second session and observed that she was able to complete them without difficulty. Much of the second session was spent working on stressful situations in which Pam could not say no to adult family members. Pam and her therapist identified her feelings in these situations and the types of thoughts and history that accompanied the feelings. Pam agreed to read Chapter 3 (Identifying and Rating Your Moods) during the following week and write down her feelings in situations in which she felt her family took advantage of her.

During the third session, the therapist helped Pam develop a list of tactful ways to say no and identify the thoughts that interfered with her practice of assertion. Pam reported some decrease in depression as a result of feeling less guilty about not meeting everyone's expectations. She also had attended an Al-Anon meeting and liked the people she met there. Pam agreed to practice saying no once during the week and read Chapters 4 (Thought Records) and 5 (Identifying Automatic Thoughts) in *Mind Over Mood* to learn more about identifying automatic thoughts. Finally, she agreed to call her husband's employee assistance program counselor to find out what treatment options would be available if her husband agreed to get help.

The next week Pam was much brighter and reported that the manual was helping her straighten out her thinking. She reported that she identified with Marissa in the book because Marissa also was depressed and, like Pam, had a history of sexual abuse. Pam said she was having some difficulty distinguishing between thoughts and feelings, although review of her worksheets showed that she only occasionally misidentified thoughts as feelings. She and the therapist discussed the differences between thoughts and feelings using Pam's worksheets as examples.

A recurrent thought was identified for situations where Pam wanted to say no but could not: "They will leave me or hurt me." This belief was examined in the session. A brief review of Pam's history, including the physical and sexual abuse she received as a child when she tried to assert herself, helped her understand where this belief originated. She and her therapist then reviewed Pam's current family (husband and adult children) and their responses to her infrequent assertiveness. She recalled that, although her current family acted angry when she asserted herself, they usually apologized within a few hours and recently had even told her that she was right to say no. This conceptualization linking her belief, her history, and her current experience was exciting to Pam. She left with more assertion plans and a commitment to read Chapter 6 (Where's the Evidence?) of the treatment manual. The fifth session was scheduled two weeks later because of the therapist's vacation.

The remaining three sessions were scheduled three weeks apart because Pam found it helpful during the two-week break to have more time for the exercises in the manual. She also wanted more time to pursue a treatment evaluation with her husband for his alcoholism, practice assertiveness, and experiment with solving her problems independently. Although Pam had many problems, the skills taught in *Mind Over Mood* and their focused application to current problems were sufficient to help her make significant progress in brief therapy. By the end of treatment Pam was able to set appropriate limits on demands made by other family members, she attended Al-Anon meetings regularly, and she no longer took responsibility for her husband's drinking. Her husband had entered and dropped out of treatment. Despite the mixture of improvements and setbacks in her life, Pam's depression had decreased. She wrote the therapist a few months later that she still had many problems but that she was making slow progress and continued to use the treatment manual.

As illustrated in this case example, when *Mind Over Mood* is used as a template for treatment, its usefulness is enhanced by a therapist who helps the client apply the skills taught to problems directly linked to the client's treatment goals. Since Pam was able to use the manual fairly independently, the therapist could accomplish additional tasks during therapy sessions. If Pam had had difficulty in learning the skills taught in *Mind Over Mood*, the therapist would have spent a greater portion of the therapy session in directly reviewing the treatment manual and the exercises completed by the client and in practicing skills.

It is important to allow the client to determine the speed with which therapy using a treatment manual can progess. The skills taught in *Mind Over Mood* build sequentially, so the client should not continue in the manual until the exercises in the current chapter can be completed with some ease and confidence. It is therefore important that the therapist review the client's worksheets from each chapter. Review allows the client the opportunity to tell the therapist what he or she is learning and to discuss some of the problem situations faced during the week and described on the worksheets. Review of worksheets also informs the therapist how well the client understands and can practice the skills described in each chapter. Later in this chapter we suggest strategies for addressing skill deficits with the client.

Using *Mind Over Mood* as an Adjunct to Treatment

Perhaps you use a therapeutic approach different from that described in *Mind Over Mood* and yet consider the skills in the client manual helpful for your clients to learn. Or you work in a setting where there is no time for psychotherapy and medication is the sole mode of treatment. Or you are permitted to do only brief crisis-oriented intervention, not enough treatment for clients who have ongoing difficulties. These are some of the circumstances in which *Mind Over Mood* can be used as an adjunct to treatment.

Even when *Mind Over Mood* is not a carefully integrated part of structured therapy, it can have therapeutic value to clients if the therapist follows a few simple steps.

- Spend time orienting the client to *Mind Over Mood*. Describe how and why you think it might be helpful. Tell the client which chapters you think will be most useful for his or her problems and in which order you recommend they be read.

- Warn the client that not all skills will be easy to apply and that patience will be needed to complete as many exercises as necessary to learn the skills in each chapter. Tell the client what help is available from you or others if difficulties are encountered.

Carlos is a physician in a health maintenance organization. He manages the medication for a large number of depressed and anxious patients. He offers his patients *Mind Over Mood* as an adjunct to medication. Patients interested in using the treatment manual are told to read specific chapters according to protocols offered in Chapters 4 and 5 of the clinician's guide.

Carlos tells his patients, "Each chapter has worksheets to complete. The worksheets will help you understand your depression/anxiety better and help you learn skills to help yourself feel better. Most people need to use the book for several months to learn these skills. It is important that you do each exercise as many times as necessary to understand it well. Some exercises you will need to do only once. Other exercises you might have to do five or even ten times before you understand them. Don't hurry through the book: use it for as many days a week as you have time.

"If you try an exercise several times and you still don't understand how to do it, reread the chapter and examples. If it still is confusing to you, we can take five minutes at our next medication check-up to see if I can help you. If I can't help you in that amount of time, I will refer you to a therapist for more help."

═══════════

• Set reasonable expectations with your client. Do you think the manual will help resolve the client's depression completely or reduce it by half? Is this a client who will be able to complete most of the chapters in a matter of weeks, or is this client likely to need a week or more for each chapter?

═══════════

Pat works in a crisis clinic. She sees many low-income clients with mood problems and borderline personality disorder who need but cannot afford more therapy than she is able to provide. She offers these clients *Mind Over Mood* and actively promotes long-term use by setting reasonable expectations for the manual's helpfulness.

"This book may help you manage some of the problems in your life. It's not a quick fix, because those don't tend to last. This is a book for you to use day by day, month to month, year after year. It may help you feel better right away, or it may not seem to help much at all. But if you stick with it, you can learn to understand your moods better and learn some ways to feel better. I recommend that you spend a week or more on each chapter until you find a chapter that really helps. Stick with that chapter for a few weeks, and then move on until you find another helpful chapter.

"When you reach the end of the book, go back and reread the chapters that helped you most. Most exercises in this book are all repeated at the back of the manual, so you can copy them and use them as many times as you need to in the years ahead. It will be up to you to read the book slowly and figure out what chapters and exercises are most helpful to you."

- Demonstrate interest in clients' use of the manual. Ask how they like the book if you see them in subsequent weeks. If you are not likely to see a client, you might ask him or her to telephone you in a few weeks with a quick progress report.

- If possible, show clients how the manual applies to their lives before sending it home. You might open to the first chapter and show how your treatment fits the model for understanding problems in Figure 1.1 on page 4. Discussion of the manual provides a bridge between the treatment you give clients and *Mind Over Mood*; clients can more easily link the approach of the manual to whatever they have already learned from you.

Bob has been using a psychodynamic approach to help Melanie with her depression. He recently learned about *Mind Over Mood* and decides to add it to her therapy because Melanie is still quite depressed. She is also on antidepressant medication.

Bob tells Melanie, "I'd like to give you a book to read and use between our therapy appointments. It describes things you can do to help your depression. Just as we added medication to your therapy, we can add this self-help manual as well. To show you how therapy, medication, and the manual fit together, let's look at the model for understanding your depression shown in Chapter 1 (*points to Figure 1.1*) of the book.

"You'll learn in this book how these five parts of your life fit together. The antidepressant you take is working to improve the physical part of your depression. In therapy, we are working to understand the connections between your past environments and your current moods, behaviors, and thoughts. The book will teach you some things you can do to change some of the negative ways you think about things when you are depressed. Some of the ideas in the book will be like the ones we talk about in therapy and some may be different. If you have any questions when you read the book, we can talk about them in here. Do you have any questions right now?"

Using *Mind Over Mood* to Develop Specific Skills

Perhaps you are seeing a couple in therapy. You want each of them to learn to identify and test their automatic thoughts when angry, but there never is enough time in the session to accomplish it. Or you work in an inpatient substance abuse program, and most of your patients can't identify feelings. Perhaps you want to help a client struggling with procrastination see the relationship between his current difficulties and core beliefs. Each of these therapy situations requires teaching clients specific skills. A third way to use *Mind Over Mood* is to identify particular skill deficits in your clients and assign the specific chapters that target the deficient skills.

The first two methods described for using *Mind Over Mood* involve total client immersion in the complete manual, with or without therapist guidance. Some clients might need to learn only one or two of the skills taught in the manual. For these clients, target chapters can be either carefully integrated into therapy or used as an adjunctive treatment according to the guidelines provided in the first two methods.

As an example, the angry couple may not need to learn to identify emotions. They can begin by reading Chapter 5 (Automatic Thoughts) in the manual. Each partner can read this chapter and try to identify one or two automatic thoughts when angry. It will take less therapy time to answer questions about this chapter and review completed exercises than to teach the concept to the couple in therapy sessions. Subsequently, the couple can read Chapters 6 (Where's the Evidence?) and 7 (Alternative or Balanced Thinking) and practice these skills inside and outside therapy.

In assigning *Mind Over Mood* to develop certain skills, the therapist should follow the guidelines in the box on page 16 of this clinician's guide to increase the likelihood that the client will use the manual. The following section discusses strategies for increasing client compliance in more detail.

STRATEGIES FOR INCREASING CLIENT COMPLIANCE

How and what we ask clients to do in therapy has a big influence on whether or not they do it. Following a few simple guidelines will greatly increase the likelihood that clients will comply with using *Mind Over Mood* in the ways you assign.

1. Make assignments small.

Reading and writing assignments should be small enough to fit in a client's schedule. For example, a working mother with two small children may have to make an enormous effort to spend even five minutes a day reading or writing. Discuss reasonable expectations with each client. Some clients may spend 15 to 20 minutes per week, others may be able to spend as much as an hour per day.

2. Assign tasks within the client's skill level.

Mind Over Mood is written to help clients develop critical skills that have been linked with improved mood and more effective problem solving. Even so, a client usually has to read a chapter more than once to learn the skill. And some chapters presuppose skills taught in earlier chapters. For example, if a client is asked to complete a Thought Record (Chapters 6 and 7) before learning to identify hot thoughts (Chapter 5), the client may not be able to complete the assignment. Use the Cognitive Therapy Skills Checklist on page 30 of this guide to assess whether a particular assignment is within a client's skill repertoire. Role-play of behavioral assignments can also be used to assess skills.

3. Make assignments relevant and interesting.

Therapy assignments should be linked to client goals and made as interesting as possible. Consider Bill, who wants greater success in his relationships. Which of these assignments do you think he would be most likely to complete? (a) Write down ten automatic thoughts this week. (b) Read Chapter 6 (Where's the Evidence?). (c) Imagine that you are preparing to call Pat for a date. Write down three automatic thoughts that might stop you from making the call. Pick one of these thoughts, read Chapter 6, and see if you can complete the evidence columns of the Thought Record using the questions in the Helpful Hints box on page 70 for guidance.

Although assignment (c) is more complex, Bill is more likely to complete it because it is relevant to his problem. Also, if calling for dates has been a roadblock for Bill, he will probably be interested to learn more about this problem area. The Helpful Hints box on Page 70 of *Mind Over Mood* could help him begin to resolve his difficulty. Therefore, Bill will benefit more from assignment (c) than from either (a) or (b), which are more rote.

4. Collaborate with the client in developing learning assignments.

Encourage clients to collaborate in selecting and planning therapy assignments. Clients can often figure out what steps need to be taken and how quickly they can take these steps. Part of planning assignments together is discussing whether the client is willing to do particular assignments. Don't ask clients to do things they are not willing to do or that you would not be willing to do yourself.

5. Provide a clear rationale for the assignment and a written summary.

Often clients are motivated to do therapy exercises but they forget what to do or why they are doing them. Once you and a client have chosen a learning assignment for the week, write it down. A written summary can include a rationale for the assignment (what is the client going to try to learn and how does this link to therapy goals?), a specific description of what the client will observe, read, write or do, and an alternate plan if the original assignment proves impossible. For example, the alternate assignment may be to write down thoughts and feelings that interfere with completion of the original assignment.

6. Begin the assignment during the session.

One of the best ways to make certain a client understands and can complete an assignment is to begin the assignment during the therapy session. For example, a client who is asked to write down automatic thoughts related to self-doubt can notice if he or she has any doubts regarding completion of this assignment. If so, the doubts can be written down as a sample of the type of thoughts that will be recorded. Beginning the assignment in the therapy session increases the client's understanding of what is expected. Further, difficulties that may interfere with completion of the assignment often emerge when the client attempts to begin the assignment (in writing, role-play, or imagination) under your guidance.

7. Identify and problem solve impediments to the assignment.

It is not enough to clearly assign a therapy task. Ask the client, "What could interfere with completing this exercise?" When asked, clients usually are able to anticipate difficulties that might interfere with assignment completion. Discussing the difficulties before the end of therapy appointments often increases the client's ability to comply with learning assignments. For example, if a client says, "I might forget," the two of you can discuss a plan for remembering. If a client says, "I'm not sure I'll have time to complete these observations this week," you can discuss whether to reduce the size of the assignment or how to prioritize observations to learn the most from whatever time your client can devote to the task.

8. Emphasize learning, not a particular desired outcome.

One goal of therapy is learning. Sometimes we learn more from undesirable outcomes than from whatever we consider success. Clients may become discouraged if a therapist seems to expect particular outcomes that do not occur. Therefore, do not specify what a client will learn. Instead, be open to whatever learning emerges from an experiment or written exercise.

To set the stage, you might say, "We've talked today about how saying what you want directly might make you feel less burdened by your friends. But we won't know if this works for you until you try it. A few times this week, try what we practiced today and notice how you feel and how your friends react. Then we can see if this idea is helpful or not." This instruction keeps the door open to both expected and unexpected results. For example, the client might find out that her friends attack her when she expresses her wishes. This outcome, although not expected, is important information that may shift the terms in which she and her therapist understand her problem. Perhaps she feels burdened by friends because they abuse her and do not respect her feelings.

It is the therapist's role to help the client learn *something* from every exercise completed. The therapist should strive to help a client learn from incomplete tasks as well. For example, a client who does not read an assigned chapter or complete an assigned worksheet might learn what life events, emotions, or beliefs are interfering with progress. Or the therapist might learn that certain aspects of the assignment were not clear to the client.

9. Show interest, and follow up in the next appointment.

Ideally, you also will be interested in what your client learns from therapy assignments. Showing your own enthusiasm encourages the client, and so does spending time in the next session discussing the client's efforts. How did the client's reading, writing, experiments, or observations contribute to learning or bring the client closer to the therapy goal(s)? Linking client assignments to therapy progress supports continued client effort.

PROBLEM SOLVING WHEN THE CLIENT DOES NOT IMPROVE

Although cognitive therapy helps most clients feel better and have greater success in solving problems, some clients do not improve even though they have shown good treatment compliance. If you are using *Mind Over Mood* and a client is not improving, consider the following factors to identify changes in the therapy that might lead to better outcomes.

Conceptualization and Diagnosis

Two common reasons clients do not improve are that the therapist has not conceptualized the problem in a helpful way and that the therapist has not made an accurate and complete diagnosis. For example, Mary was experiencing intense anxiety whenever she had flashbacks of being raped. Her therapist disregarded the rape's importance because it had happened ten years earlier and Mary had subsequently experienced years with low anxiety. The therapist conceptualized Mary's anxiety as poor relaxation skills and taught Mary controlled breathing to manage her anxiety. Mary did not improve because her anxiety was related to the trauma, not poor relaxation skills.

Many cases of faulty conceptualization are not as clear-cut as

Mary's anxiety. Most clients have multiple problems, and a conceptualization must consider which problems are primary and whether one conceptualization can explain them all.

Persons (1989) has written a book to describe case conceptualization in cognitive therapy. She emphasizes the importance of making a problem list with the client and then looking for belief(s), skill deficits, or behavioral patterns that help explain all the difficulties. In *Mind Over Mood* we suggest in Chapter 1 a five-part model for the problem list. Identifying hot thoughts (Chapter 5) and core beliefs (Chapter 9) can help you and the client develop the cognitive portion of a case conceptualization. Observing client skills and looking for behavioral patterns, environmental stressors, and biological factors help complete the conceptualization.

Accurate diagnosis is also important, especially since cognitive therapy has specific treatment plans for different diagnoses, as outlined in Chapters 4 through 7 of the clinician's guide. If a client is diagnosed with panic disorder when he or she really suffers from social phobia, the treatment plan for panic will not be helpful. Therefore, the first questions a therapist should consider when a client is not improving are "Have I properly diagnosed the client?" and "Are we conceptualizing the problems in a way that makes sense and is directly addressed by the treatment plan?"

Medication and Other Adjunctive Treatments

Sometimes medication or another adjunctive treatment is necessary to facilitate improvement. Clients who experience severe depression, obsessive–compulsive disorder, or disorienting distress often benefit more from therapy if they are also taking medication. People with agoraphobia may improve partially and then stop improving unless they also undergo couples or family therapy to address beliefs and behavioral patterns in the family system that support the agoraphobic avoidance.

Therapist Experience

No therapist is skilled in the treatment of every problem. A client's problems may be in areas in which the therapist is relatively inexperienced. Inexperience can be addressed by reading more about treatment models and methods for the problem or obtaining supervision from a therapist with expertise in the client's problem area(s). Alternatively, the client may be referred to a therapist with greater expertise.

Schema Interference

Some clients may have central schemas that interfere with treatment progress. For example, Kevin believed that he would be worthless if he followed the advice of someone else. Therefore, whenever his therapist suggested a strategy for anxiety management, Kevin either argued with the therapist or refused to try the method proposed. Kevin made no progress until this schema was directly addressed in therapy using the scale described in Chapter 9 of *Mind Over Mood*. Chapter 7 of the clinician's guide describes strategies you can use to improve treatment outcome with clients who hold schemas that interfere with therapy.

Therapy Relationship

As described on pages 6–10, a collaborative therapy relationship is an important foundation for client progress. Sometimes client improvement is superficial because the client does not feel safe in the therapy relationship. One man completed all therapy assignments but did not experience improvement in his anxiety because he did not feel safe telling the therapist his central fear: that he might be gay. For more information on the importance of the therapeutic relationship and processes for maintaining good relationships with clients, read Beck et al. (1990) and Wright and Davis (1994).

Sometimes disruptions in the therapy relationship occur because of therapist beliefs, expectations, or emotional reactions to clients. A therapist may have difficulty maintaining empathic rapport with a client who is describing a struggle that closely parallels a current life experience for the therapist. For example, one therapist sought supervision when she found it difficult to focus on the concerns of a male client who was considering divorce because the therapist's husband had recently announced that he was divorcing her. *Mind Over Mood* can provide a structured approach for therapists in identifying and evaluating their own interfering thoughts and emotions during problematic therapy sessions. Thought Records or Action Plans you complete to resolve your own problems can be reviewed with a colleague, a supervisor, or your own therapist, if you wish.

Skill Deficits

The Cognitive Therapy Skills Checklist below can be used as an assessment tool with a client who is not improving.

Cognitive Therapy Skills Checklist	*Mind Over Mood* Chapters
1. Understands the interaction between thoughts, moods, behavior, physical reactions, and environment.	1
2. Understands the relevant Chapters if there is a specific mood problem.	10 11 12
3. Understands the cognitive model.	2
4. Recognizes the connection between thoughts and moods.	2
5. Identifies moods.	3
6. Identifies automatic thoughts.	4&5
7. Identifies hot thoughts.	5
8. Identifies evidence in support of a hot thought as well as evidence that does not support the hot thought.	6
9. Generates alternative explanations to the hot thought based on the evidence collected.	7
10. Designs and implement experiments to test automatic thoughts.	8
11. Develops Action Plans to solve problems.	8
12. Experiences a mood shift as a result of Thought Records, experiments, and/or Action Plans.	7&8
13. Identifies underlying assumptions and core beliefs.	9
14. Recognizes and records evidence that is contrary to underlying assumptions and core beliefs.	9
15. Identifies new core beliefs and assumptions.	9
16. Recognizes and records evidence that is consistent with new assumptions and core beliefs.	9

From *Clinical Guide to Mind Over Mood* by Christine A Padesky with Dennis Greenberger. © 1995 The Guilford Press

The skills itemized in the checklist are generally acquired in sequential order as therapy progresses. Each skill is fully explained in the corresponding *Mind Over Mood* chapter. When a client is not improving, it is worthwhile to review the Cognitive Therapy Skills Checklist to determine which skills have been mastered and which remain to be learned. This review often pinpoints the skill and corresponding treatment manual chapter that need additional time.

A skills review should be done with the client, and it should incorporate the client's perceptions, the therapist's perceptions, and the manual worksheets and exercises completed to date. For example, a client will have considerable difficulty generating alternative explanations for a hot thought (skill 9) if the client has not previously learned to answer the "Where's the evidence?" questions (skill 8). Further, a client will be unlikely to experience a mood shift as a result of a Thought Record, experiment, or Action Plan (skill 12) if the client has not learned how to identify a hot thought (skill 7).

Refer to the Cognitive Therapy Skills Checklist when the client is not improving as expected or on an ongoing basis to insure that all skills are being developed. Some clients arrive at therapy with some partially or fully developed skills. Many clients, for example, are capable of identifying moods or thoughts when they begin therapy and may need little if any help in developing these skills.

If a client does have a skill deficit that seems to be interfering with therapy progress, it is important to point this out in a way that is both collaborative and noncritical. The following therapist—client dialogue illustrates a collaborative model for discussing skill deficits with a client.

T: You've been doing Thought Records for three weeks now and it seems to be a struggle for you without much payoff.

C: Yes, I'm not sure I like doing Thought Records.

T: What don't you like about it?

C: None of the alternative explanations I write down help me feel less anxious.

T: A few weeks ago when you were filling in just the first three columns— situation, moods, and automatic thoughts— I thought you were quite excited about this method.

C: I was. I found it really helpful to figure out what I was thinking. That made my anxiety seem less weird.

T: What happened when you started filling in the two evidence columns and then the alternative belief column?

C: I thought of lots of things that scared me even more. I can't think of much that convinces me not to be anxious.

T: That's really a helpful observation. It sounds as if it would help if you could find more evidence that your anxious thoughts aren't necessarily true. We could review the Helpful Hints box on page 70 and practice using the questions in therapy. Then you could use them outside therapy and tell me which ones seem most helpful in finding evidence that reduces your anxiety. How does that sound to you?

C: OK. That might help.

T: You don't sound very sure about that.

C: Well, I think it might help. But what if my anxious thoughts are true?

T: Good point. Maybe we should practice a second strategy at the same time.

C: What do you mean?

T: We haven't worked on Chapter 8 yet. It teaches you how to come up with Action Plans to solve problems. Maybe we also need to be developing a plan for how to handle it if some of the things you worry about come true.

C: I like that idea.

T: Do you think we can do both at once? Practice the questions in Chapter 6 and also start working on Chapter 8?

C: Yes, I think so. It would be easier if I knew I would be OK whether my anxious thought was right or wrong.

T: Let's try both strategies, then. Let's also talk about this idea that thoughts are right or wrong. Do you get the impression that I think your anxious thoughts are wrong?

C: No. I know you've said they can be a good warning system for me. But I can't help but feel they're wrong if they don't come true.

T: Tell me more about what you mean.

In this therapy dialogue we learn that the client is not able to generate alternative explanations for his hot thought that are credible to him (Cognitive Therapy Skills Checklist skill 9). After asking the client to review his experience in therapy to date, the therapist learns that the client has not really mastered skill 8, answering the question "Where's the evidence?" When the therapist proposes more practice of the section of *Mind Over Mood* that teaches the client how to develop skill 8 (the Helpful Hints box on page 70), the client raises an additional concern: "What if my anxious thoughts are true?" Skills 8 and 9 do not address this client concern, but skill 11 (making Action Plans) does. Therefore, the therapist moves both backward (review skill 7) and forward (skill 11) to collaborate with the client in solving the problem of nonimprovement in therapy.

TROUBLESHOOTING GUIDE

This chapter outlines a variety of guidelines to follow in using *Mind Over Mood* to enhance therapy. But even if you follow all the guidelines and suggestions, problems may still occur. Most chapters in the clinician's guide end with a Troubleshooting Guide that addresses some of the additional problems that can occur and describes how to use *Mind Over Mood* to help solve these difficulties.

Client Noncompliance with Therapy Requests and Assignments

It is important not to interpret clients' noncompliance with assignments as resistance to therapy. Instead, noncompliance should be approached with a problem-solving attitude. First, review the strategies for increasing client compliance on pages 24–27 to make sure you are doing everything possible to make compliance easy for your client. If you are following these therapist guidelines, then examine client factors. The two types of client factors that are important in understanding noncompliance are (1) life factors or problems that need to be solved and (2) beliefs that interfere with compliance.

Early in therapy, clients may come to a session without having done the assignment. It is not unusual for clients to explain that they forgot or didn't have time to do the assignment. It can be helpful in this situation to have clients estimate how much time they think the assignment will take. If the estimate seems greater than yours, review what is expected and perhaps begin the assignment in the session to evaluate the true time demand. If the estimate appears accurate, it may be worthwhile to develop practical, specific strategies to complete the assignments. The two most common strategies are scheduling a precise time to do assignments and doing assignments on an as-needed basis.

For many clients, scheduling a predesignated time to do assignments is helpful. Scheduling helps bring the therapy into their daily life. Further, if the designated time follows a daily activity such as brushing teeth, dinner, or a coffee break, then the daily activity becomes a cue and a reminder to do the assignment. A cue can be quite important for clients attempting to add a new habit to their life. A depressed client who is to do one Thought Record at a designated time every day can be asked to mentally review the previous 24 hours time and choose the most depressing moment as a focus for the Thought Record. One disadvantage of designating a time to do a Thought Record is that the memory of the experience may have dimmed by the time the Thought Record is written.

An alternative to the predetermined time method is the as-needed method. Some clients find it easier to do Thought Records and other assignments during or immediately following a difficult experience. These clients may prefer to take *Mind Over Mood* with them to work, carry it with them in their car, and keep it available while at home. For these clients the cue or reminder to do a Thought Record is the experience of a problematic emotion or behavior. The advantage of the as-needed method is that clients address difficulties immediately, giving themselves no time to forget details of the experience.

Therapists also need to attend to whether or not a nonsupportive family member, an abusive spouse, or other factors interfere with assignment compliance. For example, Mary did not do written assignments three weeks in a row. During the fourth session, she revealed that she was reluctant to write anything on paper at home because of her fear that her physically abusive husband would find it and become enraged. Mary and her therapist decided that it would be safer for her to come to her therapy sessions 30 minutes early, do her written assignments in the waiting room, and leave written material with her therapist. In this way, Mary could benefit from written assignments and be assured that her husband would not see what she had written.

When a person is ill and goes to a physician, the doctor may prescribe medication for the illness. The patient sets up the appointment, attends the appointment, has the prescription filled, and takes the medication. In cognitive therapy, clients are asked to be much more active and collaborative in their treatment. It is important to remember that most clients have never been involved in cognitive therapy and do not understand that they will be required to play an active role. It can be argued that what happens between therapy sessions is as important as what happens during them. Some evidence indicates that a client's compliance with assignments has prognostic implications: Clients who do assignments tend to get better faster. This explanation is often sufficient to increase compliance. It is best to provide a thorough rationale for active therapy participation along with or before the first assignment.

If a client routinely does not complete assignments, noncompliance can be a focus in therapy. Noncompliance is a valuable opportunity to discover beliefs that need to be addressed before therapy progresses. For example, consider how each of the following beliefs would affect compliance with homework: "It's hopeless; nothing I do will make a difference," "I won't do it right," "I won't do it perfectly," "My therapist will criticize me," "If I show my therapist what I am thinking she will know I'm crazy," "If my therapist really cared, she would know how tough it is for me and not ask me to do more."

It is important for therapists to look for the beliefs that accompany noncompliance and address them using the methods detailed in *Mind Over Mood*. Evaluating beliefs increases the likelihood of changing noncompliance to compliance, and it also can pinpoint underlying assumptions and core beliefs that may be contributing to other problems in the client's life. For a further discussion of core beliefs and their influence on therapy, see Chapter 7 of this guide. Chapters 6 and 9 in *Mind Over Mood* describe strategies to help clients evaluate beliefs interfering with therapy compliance.

Client Inability to Read and Write

A client who is unable to read and write cannot use *Mind Over Mood* directly. However, a therapist working with the client could use *Mind Over Mood* to guide treatment planning and client exercises. Clients who cannot read often benefit from pictorial reminders of what they are learning in therapy. For example, a client keeping a core belief record (*Mind Over Mood*, Chapter 9) could cut out and save magazine pictures to remember events that support a new core belief. The therapist could select certain pages of the treatment manual for use with a client with limited reading ability. Clients who can read but cannot write could use a tape recorder to complete *Mind Over Mood* exercises. In these ways, therapists can creatively adapt the material in *Mind Over Mood* for use with many clients who might seem poorly suited for a written treatment manual.

Other Problems

If you identify problems not addressed here in your use of *Mind Over Mood* as a cognitive therapy treatment manual, please write us. If you wish, you can send us the therapist feedback form at the end of this guide. We may be able to suggest strategies to help you resolve roadblocks in your use of *Mind Over Mood*. And with your helpful feedback, future editions of *Mind Over Mood* and this therapist guide can help an even greater number of clients.

RECOMMENDED READINGS

Beck, A.T. (1976). *Cognitive therapy and the emotional disorders.* New York: International Universities Press.

Beck, A.T. (1991). Cognitive therapy: A 30-year retrospective. *American Psychologist, 46*(4), 368–375.

Beck, J. S. (1995). *Cognitive therapy: Basics and beyond.* New York: Guilford Press.

Meichenbaum, D., & Turk, D. (1987). *Facilitating treatment adherence: A practitioner's guidebook.* New York: Plenum.

Pantalon, M.V., Lubetkin, B.S., & Fishman, S.T. (1995). Use and effectiveness of self-help books in the practice of cognitive and behavioral therapy. *Cognitive and Behavioral Practice, 2*(1), 213–228.

Persons, J. (1989). *Cognitive therapy in practice: A case formulation approach.* New York: W.W. Norton.

Teasdale, J., & Barnard, C. (1992). *Affect, cognition and change.* London: Lawrence Erlbaum Associates.

Wright, J.H., & Davis D. (1994). The therapeutic relationship in cognitive-behavioral therapy: Patient perceptions and therapist responses. *Cognitive and Behavioral Practice, 1*(1), 25–45.

2

Individualizing
MIND OVER MOOD
for Clients

One of the challenges we encountered in writing a cognitive therapy treatment manual was how to address the varied needs of individuals using the book. Some people entering therapy need to learn basic skills such as identifying emotions; others may be ready to begin testing automatic thoughts; still others need help only to solve one or two life problems. You as therapist play an important role in the individualization process. Although *Mind Over Mood* is written to build skills step by step, you may use the book fluidly, assigning chapters in a different order, assigning only a few chapters for particular clients, or using the book as a self-guided client reference. Chapters 4 through 10 of this guide suggest strategies for using *Mind Over Mood* for different client diagnoses and in different treatment settings. Other factors that will help you individualize the treatment manual to your client's needs are considered here.

INDIVIDUALIZING THE LANGUAGE
OF *MIND OVER MOOD*

It is helpful to supplement the language in *Mind Over Mood* with words, images, and metaphors from the client's life. This makes the manual more alive and enables clients to see how it applies to their life circumstances. As examples, among the four clients profiled in *Mind Over Mood*, athletic metaphors would be effective for Vic, while Marissa would respond to metaphors of survival or rebirth. The effectiveness of cognitive therapy is in large part contingent on your understanding of each of your clients and your ability to draw on appropriate language and metaphor while developing a sound therapeutic relationship. Therefore, when using the treatment manual, use individualized metaphors and personal examples from your client's life to provide additional illustrations of treatment principles.

As an example, consider Cynthia, who works in a day-care center. Her therapist describes the treatment manual as a guide to easier living: "Just as you help the children at the center learn to play with each other and get along without their parents, this book will help you learn advanced adult skills, like how to recognize your moods and thoughts and how to use this knowledge to solve your problems. It's adult mood care instead of child day care." Jack works as an auto mechanic. His therapist introduces the treatment manual as a repair guide for moods. "Just as the manuals for different makes of cars show you what to do to fix them, this book shows you what to do to fix your moods and personal problems."

SIMPLIFYING *MIND OVER MOOD*

Although most clients are capable of reading the entire treatment manual, some clients may be limited in reading ability or attention span. For example, a client who is severely depressed may have difficulty reading more than a page or two at a time. One way to simplify *Mind Over Mood* is to describe the four characters followed in the manual (Ben, Marissa, Linda, and Vic) and ask clients to pick the character who is most like them. A client can then be instructed to read *Mind Over Mood* following this one character and ignoring most of the text related to the other characters.

Suppose the seriously depressed client chooses to follow Marissa, who is also very depressed. In Chapter 1 the therapist crosses out the sections describing Vic and Linda and asks the client to read only the opening pages of the chapter (which introduce concepts via Ben, who is also depressed), the section describing Marissa, and the exercise "Understanding Your Own Problems." Eliminating the sections on Vic and Linda reduces the chapter length almost by half and also eliminates the discussion of anxiety, which the depressed client does not need at this time. The therapist can similarly trim the following chapters to help create a shorter, easier-to-read version of *Mind Over Mood* for the depressed client. The therapist should provide guidance on what to read in each chapter because some important learning points will be missed if all references to Vic and Linda are skipped.

ADAPTING *MIND OVER MOOD* TO A CLIENT'S CULTURE

The cognitive therapy skills that help in overcoming mood and behavioral difficulties seem to be the same for all clients. However, clients learn skills more easily if the skills are presented in a context congruent with clients' culturally acceptable beliefs, behaviors, and emotional expressions. Beliefs, behaviors, emotional and even physiological responses to situations vary depending on the cultural background of the client. Consider the three levels of thought described in Chapter 1: automatic thoughts, underlying assumptions, and schemas. Culture plays a powerful role in shaping each level of thought, as illustrated in the following examples.

Core beliefs, or schemas, are influenced strongly by culture. In the United States, for example, a predominant schema values individualism. Consistent with this schema, children are taught to contribute to classroom discussions, seek recognition for individual achievement, and express opinions. In the Japanese culture, this behavior is considered rude because a predominant schema for the Japanese is being part of the group. Japanese students are silent until the teacher expresses an opinion, achievement is attributed to the group, and individuals try to become as similar to others as possible.

An American therapist raised with an individualistic schema can easily misdiagnose and misunderstand a Japanese American client holding a group schema. As an example, a 30-year-old Japanese American man sought therapy for depression soon after graduating from law school. He had recently returned home to live with his parents and work in a family business. Therapists in the clinic where he sought treatment diagnosed this client as depressed with dependent personality disorder. From his therapist's perspective, the primary data supporting the personality disorder diagnosis were the man's strong desire to live with his parents and the "underachievement" entailed in working in a family store rather than practicing law. A Japanese American therapist reviewing this case diagnosed the client with adjustment disorder with depression and saw no evidence of a personality disorder. Within traditional Japanese American culture, living with one's parents and working in a family business indicate positive adjustment and good mental health (P. M. Yasuda, personal communication, January 20, 1995).

Underlying assumptions are the conditional rules or "should" statements used to guide our behavior, emotional expression, and understanding of how the world operates. They also vary greatly by culture. European Americans hold the underlying assumption "If someone approaches you with direct eye contact and a smile, the person is friendly." In some Native American cultures, this behavior is interpreted as hostile and disrespectful (Allen, 1973). It is important for therapists to be familiar with cross-cultural differences in underlying assumptions. Otherwise therapists may breach the therapy relationship by violating fundamental relationship rules or may view client beliefs as idiosyncratic when they are, in fact, normative in the client's culture.

Content of automatic thoughts also varies by culture. The cognitive model of panic, for example, suggests that panic is triggered by catastrophic misinterpretation of body or mental sensations (Clark, 1989). This theory is being examined cross-culturally and, while the model fits all cultures studied to date, the content of catastrophic automatic thoughts varies depending on cultural beliefs about body and mental sensations. For example, a European man with rapid heart rate may panic following the thought "I'm having a heart attack." A Chinese man experiencing rapid heart rate may panic with the thought "I'm haunted by an evil spirit who will kill me" (P. M. Salkovskis, personal communication, October 6, 1994).

Much more research needs to be done to document cultural influences on cognitive content and structure. This is particularly important because core beliefs influence behaviors, emotional experience, physiological reactions, and interpersonal interactions. Therapists should be aware that cultural differences exist in all these areas and that good case conceptualization includes recognition and understanding of these differences.

With a particular client, the first step in recognizing and understanding cultural influences is to listen carefully for them in what the client says. For example, a Japanese American client might say, "When I made this decision, I disappointed my parents" and look either ashamed or defiant. The statement combined with the ashamed emotional response might signal a client who accepts certain aspects of Japanese cultural values (deference to parental wishes); the defiant emotional response might signal one who is immersed in the values yet is actively rebelling against them.

Second, consider ways in which a client's culture influences the conceptualization of the client's problems and the treatment plan. Therapists can err in ignoring culture or overattributing cultural influence on problems. Therapists who do not even notice a client's race or do not inquire about religious beliefs are guilty of the first error. The second error was made by a therapist who said, "Poor people won't use a treatment manual because they are not motivated to change."

Third, therapists have a responsibility to educate themselves regarding client cultures in order to listen better and understand the context of a client's experience. A list of texts that discuss culture in the context of psychotherapy is included at the end of this chapter. Fourth, it is helpful to consult with colleagues regarding cultures new to your experience as a therapist. For example, one of the authors consulted a psychologist who was a practicing Mormon to better understand the role culture might play in the treatment of depression for a Mormon client.

Finally, therapists are encouraged to openly discuss culture with clients. It is helpful to honestly convey your knowledge or lack of understanding of a particular culture. Clients can be encouraged to give feedback if the therapy violates cultural assumptions or ignores important cultural meanings. Sometimes educating the therapist about culture can help a client clarify beliefs and values that the client may have followed for years but never articulated. However, it is not professionally responsible for the therapist to rely solely on the client for cultural education. Clients may not be aware or able to articulate cultural and (to the therapist) idiosyncratic forms of beliefs, behaviors, and emotional responses. Furthermore, clients have limited therapy time and therapists' cultural education should account for only a small allotment of the time available.

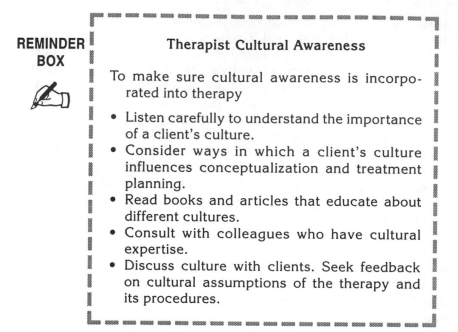

REMINDER BOX

Therapist Cultural Awareness

To make sure cultural awareness is incorporated into therapy

- Listen carefully to understand the importance of a client's culture.
- Consider ways in which a client's culture influences conceptualization and treatment planning.
- Read books and articles that educate about different cultures.
- Consult with colleagues who have cultural expertise.
- Discuss culture with clients. Seek feedback on cultural assumptions of the therapy and its procedures.

The four clients profiled in *Mind Over Mood* are drawn from our own clinical practices, which are largely made up of working- and middle-class clients voluntarily seeking therapy. You may work with clients who are impoverished, who come through court referrals, or who differ in some other way from the clients described in this manual. You can supplement the case examples in the treatment manual with examples from the lives of people similar to your clients whenever you feel it would help make the treatment manual more accessible.

We tried to use client names throughout the manual that were not associated with any one cultural or racial group. After careful consideration, we decided to minimize references to ethnicity, culture, religious affiliation, and sexual orientation. These factors are important in adapting the treatment manual to a particular client. We hoped that by excluding such factors, readers would identify with our client examples by assuming that the factors in the examples were similar to their own. You can encourage identification by suggesting that your client imagine that the characters in the book are similar to the client in race, culture, and any other group identification important to the client.

Therapeutic collaboration requires therapists to take responsibility for understanding a client's culture and adapting therapy methods to maximize client improvement within it. Four cultural factors that are important to consider in individualizing *Mind Over Mood* for clients are (1) ethnic/racial heritage, (2) socioeconomic status, (3) religious/spiritual affiliations, and (4) gender and sex-role values (Davis & Padesky, 1989). Some examples of ways you might modify use of the treatment manual to account for these cultural variations follow.

Ethnic/Racial Heritage

Ethnic and racial heritage powerfully shapes beliefs, behaviors, and life experience. Recent immigrants may emphasize or deny the importance of cultural values and behaviors to their children. Members of some racial groups are regularly devalued by others in society, whereas members of other racial groups (those with greater power and wealth) may be overvalued. Families help shape beliefs, behaviors, and emotional responses to life events, and society further endorses or punishes individual variations in response.

As an example, Vietnamese culture teaches that children should not make eye contact with adults. Children of Vietnamese families who immigrated to the United States are often instructed by teachers to make eye contact when speaking to the teacher in the classroom. Many children learn the North American value of eye contact and begin to make eye contact with parents at home. At home, eye contact is severely punished by parents wishing to raise proper sons and daughters. This parental punishment, considered good parenting within Vietnamese culture, raises concerns of child abuse in schoolteachers who are completely unaware of the role they play in creating the problem. This example illustrates how ignorance and misunderstanding of ethnic or racial cultural beliefs and behaviors can lead to unintended harm.

As therapists, we want to use *Mind Over Mood* and other therapy aids in culturally knowledgeable and sensitive ways. Following are illustrations of how you might modify use of the treatment manual according to a client's ethnic or racial background. Of course, every racial and ethnic group includes great individual variation, so these suggestions should not be applied stereotypically to all members of a particular group.

African Americans

Many African Americans have grown up in circumstances of harsh struggle with racial discrimination and economic hardship. Throughout these struggles, the African American community has provided great support and strength to its members, reflecting the African cultural value of the community over the individual (Greene, 1994). Some African American clients may therefore show little interest in an individualized treatment manual unless a bridge is built to their family and the larger community in which they live.

Clients who are strongly tied to their community may benefit more from group therapy than from individual therapy. Chapter 9 of this guide describes using *Mind Over Mood* with groups. African American clients may participate more readily in therapy groups including other African Americans than in groups predominantly composed of clients from other races. For example, Hatch and Paradis (1993) describe a group cognitive therapy treatment for panic disorder offered to a small group of African American women. These women reported that it was helpful to meet other African Americans with similar problems who had been helped.

While the clients in the Hatch and Paradis group suggested that it would be helpful to have a self-help book because audiovisual material makes it easier to understand treatment principles, they noted the absence of African American role models in written and video materials. For such clients, it would be helpful to identify characters in *Mind Over Mood* as African American or to discuss how their community experiences are similar or different from those described in the book. For example, when Marissa receives warnings from her supervisor that could lead to being fired from her job (*Mind Over Mood*, Chapter 8), African American clients may be sensitized to weigh Marissa's job performance deficiencies with possible racism that might influence the supervisor's feedback or the burdens Marissa feels in the workplace.

Another way to include community in the therapy of African American clients is to conduct cotherapy with two or more family members or neighbors. One of the authors conducted cotherapy with an African American brother and sister (both in their twenties) who both suffered from panic attacks with agoraphobia. *Mind Over Mood* was not written when this therapy was conducted, but these clients could have used it to guide discussion with each other and to keep a record of the therapy steps they followed. These two young adults benefitted from mutual encouragement throughout the therapy and created a therapeutic support community of two. African American group members in the Hatch and Paradis study cited use of positive family networks as an important aid in overcoming panic.

Many African Americans are subjected to chronic racism throughout their lives. It is important that therapists keep this environmental context in mind when teaching clients to do Thought Records. For example, one African American client came to therapy for help with anxiety. He chronically feared being fired from his job. At first, his Anglo American therapist thought his fear was purely a catastrophic distortion. Direct evidence listed on his Thought Records regarding this fear (*Mind Over Mood*, Chapter 6) showed that he had an above-average work performance and that his job performance was not being directly questioned by his supervisors.

However, the client was the only non-Anglo worker in a work force of 150. In time, the therapist came to understand the origins of his fears as subtle negative comments from coworkers were discussed and a life history of racism was explored. While this man was not likely to be fired outright—there were no performance deficiencies to justify such action by the employer—the therapist eventually agreed with the client that he would be vulnerable if the company needed to reduce its work force. The client's anxiety decreased when the therapist shifted therapeutic tactics to developing an Action Plan (*Mind Over Mood*, Chapter 8) to protect the client's job and find a new job if the current job were lost. Discounting the risk of job loss in the absence of evidence was not a reasonable therapeutic stance for this client.

Hispanic or Latino Culture

The words *Hispanic* and *Latino* describe the diverse cultures of people from Spain, Mexico, South America, Central America, Cuba, and Puerto Rico and their descendants born in other countries. While there are important differences among the geographical groups, they share a strong emphasis on commitment to family, meaning extended family. Common themes that emerge in therapy with Latino clients include concerns about interpersonal conflict in the family, a tendency to hold in anger when upset rather than to express it, and cultural prohibitions against asking for help (Organista, Dwyer, & Azocar, 1993).

Clients who share these values might be critical of the angry outbursts of Vic in *Mind Over Mood*. These segments of the book could be used to discuss cultural differences in the expression of anger. Latino clients could suggest ways Vic could tone down his anger while still communicating with Judy, his wife. It is important that Latino clients learn to express anger in ways congruent with their culture. For example, Latino clients might need to practice calm, tactful assertion as a way of increasing anger expression rather than reducing anger outbursts. Vic might be an image of how a Latino client fears he or she will appear while expressing anger. Clients can be urged to find a culturally acceptable middle ground between silent anger and Vic's explosive outbursts.

Time spent building a personal relationship is particularly important in the therapy of members of Latino cultures. Rather than presenting *Mind Over Mood* to a Latino client in the opening session of therapy, it is better to focus on establishing a relationship first. The manual can be presented later, in a warm manner. For example, you might say, "There are a number of things you can learn to help you feel better. I will help you learn some of these things, and I recommend a book that can teach you in between our meetings. By using the book to learn new ways to handle your problems, we will have more time to talk about your family and other important parts of your life when we meet together."

Cultural prohibitions against seeking help can be addressed by presenting *Mind Over Mood* as a teaching text. Working with a group of unmarried Puerto Rican mothers, Comas-Diaz (1981) introduced cognitive–behavioral therapy as a classroom activity to reduce the stigma of seeking help. These groups also encouraged personal small talk to familiarize group members with each other and build trust in a familylike atmosphere. Of course, *Mind Over Mood* can be used only with Latino clients fluent in English.

Asian Americans

Like the word *Latino*, the term *Asian American* denotes a wide mix of cultural backgrounds including Chinese, Filipino, Indian, Japanese, Korean, Pacific Islander, and Southest Asian. These cultures vary so much that the word *Asian* is virtually meaningless (Bradshaw, 1994). Therefore, the following clinical suggestions should be followed only if the ideas are compatible with the background, beliefs, and values of a particular Asian American client.

Iwamasa (1993) notes that cognitive–behavioral therapy is well-suited culturally to Asian American clients, who often prefer structured and directive therapies. Unlike Latino clients who may not return to therapy unless a relationship is carefully established, Asian American clients may not return to therapy unless the presenting problem is addressed directly and some progress is evident in the first session (Sue & Zane, 1987). Asian American clients may therefore welcome receipt of a treatment manual in the first session. Assignments from *Mind Over Mood* can reassure Asian American clients that their presenting problems will be addressed in a structured and straightforward fashion.

Focusing on client thoughts (*Mind Over Mood*, Chapters 4–9) rather than feelings (*Mind Over Mood*, Chapter 3) may be more helpful and comfortable for Asian-American clients (Iwamasa, 1993). While awareness of emotions is very important in cognitive therapy, some Asian American clients may choose to be more private about their emotional reactions than about their thoughts. Thus, while Chapter 3 and Chapters 10 through 12 of *Mind Over Mood*, which describe emotional reactions and their cognitive themes, may be of great interest to Asian American clients to read, the depth of discussion of these chapters with the therapist will vary according to client comfort.

Many of the religious philosophies of Asian-American cultures—Confucianism, Buddhism, Hinduism, Islam—include teachings about the interactive role of events, emotions, and thoughts in people's lives that may counter implicit assumptions in *Mind Over Mood*. For example, Buddhism includes a nonlinear view of life events. Therefore, a Buddhist reading case examples in *Mind Over Mood* would consider the developmental history of the example clients' problems unimportant; causality is not an issue in Buddhist philosophy (DeVos, 1980).

Collaboration with clients can include asking whether anything taught in the treatment manual is contrary to religious beliefs or personal/cultural understandings of mind, body, and event interactions. Where differences exist, client and therapist should construct a mutual understanding of learning principles taught in the treatment manual that are consistent with client beliefs and values. For example, an Asian client who enters therapy to strengthen the willpower to endure painful thoughts (Sue, 1981) may see sections of *Mind Over Mood* that teach clients to change negative thoughts rather than endure them as a weak route to better mental health. Advantages of cognitive change more compatible with Asian culture can be emphasized, such as the value of seeing the whole (positive, neutral, and negative) instead of just the parts (negative only).

Hindu Indian clients often believe in the concepts of dharma, which pertains to one's place and role in life (which one would not aspire to change), and karma, which describes a cycle of reincarnation in which one's deeds in this life determine one's form in the next life. These beliefs may conflict with "Western concepts of psychotherapy, which stress looking within or taking personal responsibility for one's own life experiences" (Jayakar, 1994, p. 178). Advice is more comfortable than self-examination for many Indian clients.

Therefore, *Mind Over Mood* could be presented to them as a guide-book.

The therapist should regularly assess with an Indian client whether or not the ideas presented in *Mind Over Mood* seem sensible and fitting with the client's beliefs, and differences in view should be discussed. It may be beneficial to assess whether the change methods described in *Mind Over Mood* could be used to improve behavior and thus improve one's karma. For example, an Indian who is depressed may be less capable of caring well for children or performing work tasks, and improvement in child care or job performance (behavior) may be more important to the client than relief from depression. Therefore, you might want to emphasize using *Mind Over Mood* for learning to improve functioning.

Middle Eastern Clients

In Middle Eastern cultures, people are highly identified with the behavior of ancestors several generations in the past. One therapist described a client who experienced chronic depression partly maintained by the negative schema "I'm bad." This schema related not to any particular deficiencies in the client but to multigenerational family shame following theft committed by the client's great-grandfather. To help this man, the therapist modified the Historical Test of Core Beliefs (*Mind Over Mood*, Worksheet 9.9) to include examination of the family history of many of the man's ancestors.

Western therapist biases about Middle Eastern culture can lead to therapeutic impasse. One therapist began to treat an Iranian woman in traditional black-veiled garb who was seeking help for depression. The therapist believed that the black veil represents the oppression of Middle Eastern women and that treatment of depression would necessarily entail "liberating" the woman from damaging cultural values. Fortunately, a colleague who was Iranian herself told the therapist that the black veil is a source of pride, not oppression, to many traditional Iranian women. With supervision, the therapist proceeded without invalidating the client's culture.

Socioeconomic Status

Clients' socioeconomic status (SES) can influence your choices of when and how to use *Mind Over Mood* in therapy. Clients of lower economic means generally welcome a book that may reduce the cost of therapy by providing written help at home. Often, clients with lower SES face daily struggles for survival, and a treatment manual can help them maintain a problem-solving focus (*Mind Over Mood*, Chapter 8) in the face of daily challenges. It is especially important for these clients to look at the environmental contributions to problems (*Mind Over Mood*, Chapter 1) so that they do not internalize their economic problems as proof of personal deficiencies.

Therapists working with clients from lower SES backgrounds should resist, on the other hand, attributing all emotional difficulties to financial hardship. Depression and anxiety do not need to accompany financial struggle or even poverty. Also, while anger is often functional in times of hardship, its expression should be designed to help, not harm, the individual, family, and community.

Many therapists associate the reading and writing involved in using a manual such as *Mind Over Mood* with middle-class and well-educated clients. This is a therapist bias. Clients with poorer economic or educational backgrounds are quite willing to participate in cognitive therapy and do written assignments. Therapists may need to encourage clients with poor writing ability by making it clear that there are no "right" answers, the writing exercises are not tests, and spelling is not important. If clients are assured that everything they read and write in the manual is intended to help them learn and remember helpful ideas, they will be much more likely to comply with written assignments.

Sometimes people of lower SES have patterns of irregular attendance at therapy appointments. If the therapist assumes that absence indicates low motivation or resistance to therapy, both therapist and client may experience decreased motivation to work together. In fact, people with lower income often miss therapy appointments because of economic hardship (e.g., no money for bus fare), unreliable child care, or even unanticipated changes in bus schedules. Some clinics find that providing free bus tokens makes therapy more accessible to low-income clients (Miranda & Dwyer, 1993). It is also helpful to make a plan for continuing progress in therapy even when appointments are missed. *Mind Over Mood* can provide therapy continuity in the absence of weekly sessions.

Some high-income clients may object to using a treatment manual because they expect individualized attention in therapy. In these cases, the therapist can point out that the manual enhances the individualized approach to therapy because each person uses it in his or her own way. Also, the client may be more willing to use a treatment manual if informed that the skills taught in *Mind Over Mood* have been linked to better treatment outcome and lower relapse (Jarrett & Nelson, 1987; Neimeyer & Feixas, 1990; Teasdale & Fennell, 1982).

Religious/Spiritual Affiliations

Some examples of how therapists use the treatment manual in ways that respect religious beliefs were discussed in the section on ethnic/racial heritage. At times, clients express concern that the treatment manual or other therapy interventions might conflict with religious teachings. In fact, cognitive therapy is compatible with religious beliefs as long as the therapist is sensitive to and helps the client explore fears that therapy will be inconsistent with religious faith.

As an example, one woman entered therapy for help with depression, panic, and agoraphobia. She was a fundamentalist Christian and, while her physician had recommended that she see a cognitive therapist, her pastor warned members of his church that most psychologists are "anti-Christian." Therefore, the woman expressed concern in the initial phone call that her Christian beliefs would be questioned in therapy. Her therapist assured her that her religious beliefs would be respected. The therapist was careful to do so in two primary ways.

Some of the woman's beliefs that maintained her depression and anxiety were somewhat linked to her religious instruction. For example, she was harshly critical of herself for sins committed during her lifetime. Her church leader preached frequently about the horror of sin and how disappointing sinners were to God. Her therapist taught her to evaluate her self-condemnation following some of the suggestions in the Helpful Hints box on page 70 in *Mind Over Mood* and showed her how to frame the questions within her religious beliefs. Particularly helpful questions included "If God loves me [a belief consistent with her religion], then what would He say to me about these sins?" "Would God understand my sins any differently than the preacher or another human?" "Are there any ways I have been a good Christian that I am discounting and yet might count for something with God?" The woman's Christian beliefs in forgiveness and redemption as well as New Testament stories about Christ forgiving sinners were also discussed in therapy, followed by a marked lessening of her depression and anxiety.

Second, the woman acknowledged that she used prayer as a primary means of coping with anxiety. Her therapist endorsed prayer as a meaningful and useful strategy for coping with anxiety and taught her other strategies for managing anxiety (*Mind Over Mood*, Chapter 11) as well. Although it was not necessary in the therapy for this woman, sometimes it is helpful to consult religious leaders in the community to enlist their support in helping a client overcome guilt-related beliefs. For example, a young girl who became suicidal after a sexual assault by her brother received great consolation after a visit with a priest, who assured her that she had not committed a sin and was not to blame for the assault.

A Mormon woman sought therapy for depression and expressed a number of conflicting beliefs related to the religious teachings of her church. She wanted to be a good Mormon but could not reconcile herself to disagreeing with a number of church teachings. Her therapist consulted a Mormon psychologist who explained to the therapist many teachings of the Mormon church relevant to the woman's concerns. The Mormon psychologist also normalized some of the doctrinal disagreements and suggested that the therapist ask the woman if there were other Mormons who shared her questions about certain aspects of doctrine. The client was aware of like-minded individuals in her church, although it never had occurred to her to seek out these people and inquire how they had reconciled their disagreements with doctrine they agreed to follow. This intervention helped the woman achieve a satisfactory balance between her faith and her individual needs and values.

Gender and Sex-Role Values

Some have argued that gender itself is a culture, profoundly influencing beliefs, behaviors, and emotional reactions (Beall & Sternberg, 1993; Davis & Padesky, 1989). Certainly gender-determined roles can influence a client's expectations for what can be achieved in therapy. One man sought therapy to handle emotion better. In fact, he wanted to stop having emotions because he judged his anxiety "unmanly." Understanding the cognitive model of anxiety as described in Chapter 11 of *Mind Over Mood* helped him understand his reactions as normal responses to the threat and danger he felt in interpersonal situations. The cognitive model intrigued him to identify his catastrophic thoughts, which in turn helped make his anxiety less mysterious and frightening to him.

A 45-year-old woman felt stuck in her life because she was unhappy in her marriage, and yet she felt helpless whenever she imagined being single because of the belief "A husband is necessary to fix life's problems." A series of Action Plans (*Mind Over Mood*, Chapter 8) helped her evaluate her belief and claify the options. She constructed plans to cope with various situations she believed required a husband's help, such as fixing a flat tire, fixing broken appliances, and mowing the lawn. Once she had actions plans for managing these problems herself, she practiced several repairs and also successfully received help from both women friends and repair professionals on the few occasions when her own efforts failed.

Therapists should examine their own cultural biases regarding gender. Often we are not aware of our own gender-based beliefs. For example, at one workshop on gender and schema change, therapists used the worksheets in Chapter 9 *Mind Over Mood* to identify their own beliefs about male and female clients. One therapist was surprised to discover that she had different schemas regarding the male and female addicts she treated: "Male addicts are screwed-up people." "Female addicts are suffering and need my help." It was not difficult for her to identify ways in which these beliefs led to differences in her therapy with men and women.

Language can reflect or trigger gender assumptions. For example, Thought Records in most cognitive therapy texts use terms such as *irrational thought* and *rational response*. In Western culture, men are often seen as "more rational" than women and woman as "more emotional" than men. Some women react negatively to Thought Records written in terms of rationality because they see the language of rationality as attacking emotional reactions and requiring them to be like men (more rational).

Mind Over Mood minimizes gender bias in language. In *Mind Over Mood* we do not use the term *rational* in referring to beliefs. Instead we refer to *more balanced* or *alternative* thinking. This change in terms is friendly to both genders and also is more consistent with the empirical nature of cognitive therapy. That is, if a client has an automatic thought that accompanies distress, it is not empirical to assume that this thought is irrational. Instead, it is to the client's advantage to explore all the data both supporting and contradicting the thought and then evaluate the thought. Sometimes distressing thoughts describe the data well, and sometimes there is an alternative or more balanced view which describes the data even better.

Sexual orientation provides another gender-based dimension of culture. Lesbians and gay men have their own cultures and live in a majority heterosexual culture in which many hold core beliefs opposite to lesbian and gay perceptions of reality. Attaining and maintaining a positive lesbian or gay identity in a culture that often devalues or does not recognize same gender relationships can be a challenge (Padesky, 1989).

Lesbian and gay clients do not require a change in format for using the treatment manual, but it is helpful to encourage lesbian and gay clients to see themselves in the clients profiled in the book. Linda and Marissa are single and could be lesbian. While the two male clients profiled in the treatment manual are married, they can easily be imagined in relationships with men instead of women. These comparisons can be used to generate discussions of how clients perceive their own experiences as similar or different from the client examples in the treatment manual.

Chapter 2 of *Mind Over Mood*, for example, describes a luncheon in which coworker Juan begins to compliment and perhaps flirt with Marissa, who is depressed. This chapter discusses how Marissa discounts positive feedback from Juan and does not accurately read his overtures. Lesbian and gay clients might react quite differently to this example compared to heterosexual clients. Perhaps Marissa is lesbian and does not want to "come out" at work. She may not feel comfortable directly telling Juan she is not interested in dating him or any man, so she pretends to not notice his attraction to her. Gay and lesbian experience includes these types of social interactions within heterosexual culture where "misperceptions" are used for positive self-protection. Therapists can follow guidelines offered in the Reminder box on page 42 of this clinician's guide to increase awareness of gay and lesbian culture.

TROUBLESHOOTING GUIDE

A problem you may encounter in trying to apply the guidelines outlined in this chapter follows. Clinical dialogue is provided to demonstrate how the problem can be solved using therapy principles outlined in Chapters 1 and 2 of the clinician's guide.

Client Refusal to Discuss Cultural Background

While most clients are happy to describe their culture, some may be guarded or even angry if the therapist raises this issue. First, examine the manner in which you made your inquiry. Was there anything condescending or judgmental in your tone or language?

Consider the difference between "Tell me what it was like growing up black in St. Louis in the 1950s." and "Do you think you're feeling this way because you're an African American?" The first request is a request to understand the client's background, including race. The second question could be heard as belittling a client's reactions or emotions as racial stereotypes.

Second, consider the nature of your relationship with the client. Most clients are comfortable discussing their background and culture once a trusting relationship is established. Perhaps you introduced questions about culture too early in the therapy relationship. If you have a good relationship with the client and he or she responds angrily when you ask about culture, it is important to discover the meaning the question has for the client. Perhaps the client worries that discussion of culture will create distance in your relationship by accentuating differences between the two of you or by activating prejudices you might hold. Alternatively, the client may find your question naive and be irritated that you are not as knowledgeable as he or she thought you were. The following dialogue illustrates one possible therapeutic response.

T: What was it like growing up black in St. Louis in the 1950s?

C: (*Angrily*) I'm not going to talk to you about that!

T: You seem angry. Did my question offend you in some way?

C: No. But I'm sick and tired of having to educate white therapists about the black experience. What do *you* think it was like?

T: I imagine it was tough. I can even guess some of the experiences you might have had. But I don't want to assume anything because I know different people have different experiences, and I want to make sure I accurately understood yours.

C: (*In a sarcastic tone*) Yeah, I'm sure.

T: You say you're tired of educating white therapists. Have you had to do it a lot?

C: Yes. Once I spent seven weeks telling a student therapist at a clinic about what it was like for me, and then she just left because her time was up. She hadn't even told me that she was only going to be there a few months. I spent all my time helping her and didn't get any help back.

T: That would make me angry, too. What have been your other therapy experiences?

C: Another therapist felt he knew all about the black experience from some course he had taken in college. He actually corrected me on my understanding of civil rights progress. And the last therapist kept asking over and over again, "What's that like as a black man?" Like that was all I was to her—black.

T: I understand now why you are angry. You don't want to spend your time educating me or listening to my prejudices or feeling like I'm seeing you as black only.

C: That's right.

T: Well, I don't want to do any of those things, either. At the same time, I do like to ask all my clients what it was like growing up. Being black has probably been a big part of growing up for you. I bet your past experiences affect your feelings, beliefs, and re-actions to things that happen today. I might misunderstand if you don't tell me anything about it. How could we work this out?

C: I don't mind telling you about my life. I just don't want a bunch of white guilt or overreaction.

T: Give me an example of what you mean.

C: I went through some violent, awful stuff in St. Louis and watched my family go through worse. But we have come to terms with this. I don't want to help you come to terms with it. That is your own work to do. Not here.

T: So when you tell me these things, would you prefer I not ex-press sympathy, just listen and ask about your reactions and how you handled them?

C: Exactly right.

T: So let me summarize my understanding. We'll talk about your past, but only if it's linked to your current problems and can help you, not for my education or curiosity. When you tell me things, I will not express a lot of sorrow or sympathy because you've worked these things through and my sympathy will seem like "white guilt" to you.

C: You got it.

T: Two more questions. I usually do feel and express sorrow when I hear painful things people have experienced. So, will you un-derstand if I look sorrowful that this is my reaction and that I will deal with it— you don't have to?

C: Fair enough.

T: Second, how will I know if you do want to have support in looking at some of your feelings and reactions to events in your life? You know sometimes you want to avoid feelings now, and when I push you, you discover it helps to sort them out.

C: That's true. Well, you can ask me if I'm avoiding or if it's really right to move on to something else. I'll be honest with you.

T: OK. Let's try this out today. It helps me to know where you stand and why. I would like to check a few times in the next few sessions to see how you feel I'm doing in following the guidelines we've come up with. And if I step on your toes, you let me know.

C: Oh, I will! (*Laughs.*)

T: (*Laughing*) I'm sure you will. (*Pauses.*) Now, how about telling me what it was like growing up black in St. Louis in the 1950s? Tell me whatever parts you think are relevant to the anxiety you are feeling now.

The therapist asks for and listens carefully to the reasons for the client's anger. She explains clearly her views of the importance of his history for therapy. Relevant feelings, events, and beliefs are identified and summarized. Next, she collaborates with the client to devise a plan for discussing his background in ways that will help rather than harm him and the therapy relationship. Finally, they agree to evaluate their plan over time and the therapist indicates her openness to negative feedback from the client if she is not helping him in the ways discussed. The therapist and client resolve the potential roadblock following the principles of collaboration and guided discovery described in Chapter 1 of this guide.

RECOMMENDED READINGS

Beall, A.E., & Sternberg, R.J. (1993). *The psychology of gender*. New York: Guilford Press.

Comas-Diaz, L., & Greene, B. (Eds.). (1994). *Women of color: Integrating ethnic and gender identities in psychotherapy*. New York: Guilford Press.

Davis, D., & Padesky, C. (1989). Enhancing cognitive therapy with women. In A. Freeman, K.M. Simon, L.E. Beutler, & H. Arkowitz (Eds.). *Comprehensive handbook of cognitive therapy* (pp. 535–557). New York: Plenum Press.

Garnets, L., Hancock, K.A., Cochran, S.D., Goodchilds, J., & Peplau, L.A. (1991). Issues in psychotherapy with lesbians and gay men: A survey of psychologists. *American Psychologist, 46*(9), 964–972.

Hays, P.A. (1995) Multicultural applications of cognitive-behavior therapy. *Professional Psychology: Research and Practice, 25* (3), 309–315.

McGoldrick, M., Pearce, J.K., & Giordano, J. (Eds.). (1982). *Ethnicity and family therapy.* New York: Guilford Press.

Persons, J.B. (Ed.). (1993, October). Understanding diversity [Special issue]. *the Behavior Therapist, 16* (9).

Ponte, J.A., Rivers, R.Y., & Wohl, J. (1995). *Psychological interventions in cultural diversity.* Boston: Allyn Bacon.

Ridley, C. (1995). *Overcoming unintentional racism in counseling and therapy.* Thousand Oaks, CA: Sage Publications.

Sue, D. (1991). *Counseling the culturally different: Therapy and practice.* New York: Wiley.

Setting Therapy Goals

The Lewis Carroll story *Alice in Wonderland* describes a moment when Alice, facing a fork in the road, meets the Cheshire cat and asks him which road to take. The cat asks Alice where she is going. Alice, who has never been to Wonderland before, says, "I'm not really sure." The Cheshire cat then happily exclaims, "Well, then it doesn't really matter which way you go!"

Just as Alice had never been in Wonderland, many clients have never been in cognitive therapy and don't know what to expect or where they want to be at the end of therapy. To make the best use of therapy time, where you are going does matter. Helping the client set goals is therefore an important task. Once client and therapist agree on goals and the road to be taken to reach the goals, therapy can be quicker and more effective.

One of the four clients profiled in *Mind Over Mood* is Vic, a recovering alcoholic with low self-esteem, anxiety, anger, and relationship problems. Figure 3.1 shows the goals Vic and his therapist specified in the second therapy session.

Notice that Vic set general goals and also smaller, more specific goals. General goals help establish the areas of a client's life that need improvement. Specific goals itemize observable and reason-

General goals	Small specific goals
Be a better husband.	Yell less. Don't slam things. Kiss Judy good-bye. Hug Judy when I come home. Come home on time.
Stay sober.	Don't drink. Don't go out with Pete if tired. Call AA sponsor when it's hard. Go to AA meetings when traveling.
Feel calmer.	Learn how to relax in tense times. Figure out what triggers tension.
Be more successful on my job.	Call five customers a day. Get reports in on time. Talk with boss once a week.
Feel more worthwhile.	Stop kicking myself for mistakes. Learn to see my good points. Learn to accept my imperfections.

FIGURE 3.1. Vic's therapy goals.

able changes so both therapist and client can regularly monitor whether or not progress is being made.

Setting goals can be much more difficult than it appears. The Helpful Hints box on pages 60–61 provides questions you can ask your client to evaluate whether the general goals chosen are likely to be achieved in therapy. After each question are a few examples of how you might present a rationale for each question to your client. You can use these explanations directly or create your own explanations, adapting language and metaphors that will individualize goal setting for clients as described in Chapter 2 of the clinician's guide.

**HELPFUL
HINTS**

Questions to Ask Client About General Goals, with Rationales

1. Do these goals involve changing things about you?

Your goals should not involve changing other people. For example, if you set a goal to have your boyfriend stop criticizing you, this is a goal for his behavior, not your own. You have no direct control over his behavior, although you can tell him how you feel and ask him to stop.

If his criticism is a problem for you, your goals might be first to decide whether to continue the relationship that hurts you and, if you decide to stay in the relationship, to learn ways to cope with his criticism and talk with him about it.

2. Do these goals involve changing things that are in your control?

Similarly, you should not set goals that are not in your control. For example, if somebody else decides job promotions where you work, a goal to become manager of your department is not really under your control. If you want to be manager, you might set goals such as improving your work performance and meeting with your supervisor to clarify what performance standards you need to achieve to be considered for promotion.

Setting goals that are under your control means that you have a good chance of reaching them. In the work example, you can probably find out what expectations your supervisor has for the department manager and you can probably meet them. Hopefully, you will feel a sense of satisfaction as you improve your job performance. However, a manager position may not become available or a relative of the company's owner may be appointed to the position despite your best efforts.

3. Are your goals realistic?

Some goals would be nearly impossible for anybody to achieve. For example, a goal of being a millionaire by the end of the year if you currently have no savings and a job that barely pays the bills is probably not realistic.

Most of us wouldn't set a goal like this, but we often do set goals that are equally unrealistic. For example, some people who are anxious set a goal "never to feel nervous again." Since all people feel nervous sometimes in some situations, this is not a realistic goal. It would be more realistic to set such goals as "to get only as nervous as the average person," "to be able to fly in an airplane without having a panic attack," and "to get over a fear of public speaking." These are realistic and achievable goals.

Similarly, it can be unrealistic to stop all negative thoughts. If you want to be less self-critical, for example, you could set goal such as "To criticize myself less" or "To give myself as much credit for my successes as I give for my mistakes." It is unlikely that you will be able to completely stop being self-critical; all of us are self-critical sometimes—and that can be good for us in small doses.

The Helpful Hints box on page 62 lists questions that you can ask your client to help determine specific goals to measure progress. Choose the questions that seem most helpful for a particular client and a particular general goal. For example, if a client has a general goal that is vague ("I want to feel better"), questions 4, 6, and 8 might be particularly helpful in clarifying desired therapy outcomes.

HELPFUL HINTS

Questions to Ask Client to Help Set Specific Goals

1. What small steps would show that you were inching toward the goal?

2. What do you need to do first before the final goal is possible?

3. How many weeks or months do you think it will take to reach your goal? What one or two things should you do first?

4. What would be the first sign that you are making progress?

5. If this were a friend's goal, what would you advise him or her to do to get started?

6. Are there one or two smaller changes that would make you feel better and let you know you are on the right track?

7. Have you broken your goal into a number of smaller steps?

8. Are your specific goals observable? How will you know if you're making progress? What will be different in your life?

SETTING GOALS FOR EMOTIONAL CHANGE

Many clients come to therapy with the general goal of wanting to feel less depressed or less anxious. It is important to help clients break down these general emotional objectives into specific, measurable goals. The *Mind Over Mood* Depression Inventory (Worksheet 10.1) and the *Mind Over Mood* Anxiety Inventory (Worksheet 11.1) assess specific, measurable symptoms of depression and anxiety. These inventories are included in the client treatment manual to make it easy for you and the client to establish a baseline and to track overall changes from session to session. Further, the inventories allow you to assess the effectiveness of different interventions. For example, if a client scheduled pleasurable activities during the week and doing them coincided with a decrease in his or her *Mind Over Mood* Depression Inventory score, you can discuss and further evaluate whether this therapeutic intervention was responsible for the decrease in the depression.

In addition, the *Mind Over Mood* Inventories allow you and your clients to identify specific symptoms of depression and anxiety that may respond to targeted interventions. For example, suicidal thoughts, sleep disturbances, and avoidance behavior may require special attention and planned interventions. By detailing and measuring specific symptoms, you ensure thoroughness and improve the likelihood of therapeutic success.

Clients who are depressed or anxious should be instructed to complete *Mind Over Mood* Depression and Anxiety Inventories immediately before each therapy session, as described in the next two chapters of this guide. The scores should then be recorded on *Mind Over Mood* Worksheets 10.2 and 11.2 to track progress.

The general goal of some clients will be to experience an emotion less frequently. For example, one of Vic's general goals was to be angry less often and not to explode in anger at his wife. At the beginning of therapy, Vic tracked how many times per week he experienced anger and yelled at his wife. He and his therapist monitored and recorded these episodes in order to establish a baseline, set goals, and track progress.

PRIORITIZING GOALS AND TRACKING PROGRESS

Once therapy goals are specified, you and the client can decide how many goals can be accomplished in the time available. If you are doing very brief therapy with only a few meetings, probably only one or two goals can be achieved. Even if therapy is long, goals must be prioritized to decide what to work on first. In cognitive therapy, client and therapist discuss goals and determine their priority collaboratively. The Helpful Hints box on the following page suggests questions to help your client choose the highest priority goal(s).

Questions 1 and 2 help identify urgent goals. Question 3 asks the client to consider whether reaching the urgent goals depends on the accomplishment of another goal. For example, Vic may need to stay sober in order to accomplish his other goals.

If no goals are particularly urgent, you can then ask the client question 4. Question 5 considers which goal would be the easiest to achieve. The easiest goal is a good place to start if no goal is urgent or more important. Also, if your client is feeling particularly overwhelmed or hopeless, the easiest goal might seem like a manageable starting point. Accomplishing some goal, even an easy one, can increase your client's hopefulness.

Once therapy goals are established, you and your client can spend part of each session assessing progress toward the goals. As

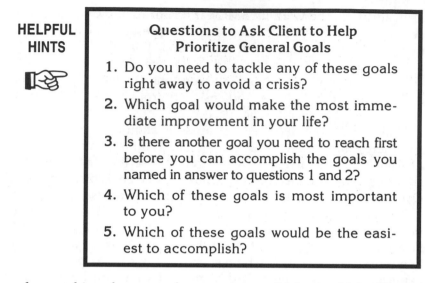

HELPFUL
HINTS

**Questions to Ask Client to Help
Prioritize General Goals**

1. Do you need to tackle any of these goals right away to avoid a crisis?

2. Which goal would make the most immediate improvement in your life?

3. Is there another goal you need to reach first before you can accomplish the goals you named in answer to questions 1 and 2?

4. Which of these goals is most important to you?

5. Which of these goals would be the easiest to accomplish?

goals are achieved, new goals can emerge as highest priority. If your client is not making progress toward achieving goals, (a) consider breaking specific goals into even smaller steps, (b) search for what is interfering with progress toward goals (e.g., thoughts, emotions, skill deficits, life circumstances), and (c) discuss with your client what could be changed or added to therapy to speed up improvement.

REMINDER
BOX

Setting Therapy Goals

- Goals help identify what clients want to change, guide plans for change, and provide guideposts to track progress.
- Breaking general goals into specific goals simplifies the change process by providing a step-by-step plan for achieving general goals.
- Prioritizing goals helps decide which goals to work on first to benefit most from therapy.
- Charting emotional changes helps monitor progress. You can track changes in emotional intensity and frequency and in specific mood-related symptoms.
- If the client is not making progress toward goals, consider breaking goals into even smaller steps, problem solve what is interfering with goal progress, or consider changes in the therapy plan.

TROUBLESHOOTING GUIDE

While the principles of goal setting are easy, this stage of therapy is difficult for many clients and therapists. Clients and therapists who do not set goals in other areas of their lives often have difficulty learning to do so in therapy, when emotional distress is often high. The following clinical examples model therapeutic responses to two common pitfalls in goal setting.

Vague Client Goals or Client Difficulty Describing Goals

The questions in the Helpful Hints box on page 62 are intended to help a client become more specific about vague goals. The following therapy excerpt illustrates this process.

T: Judy, you say you want to be a better mother. What do you mean by that?

J: I'm not sure. I just don't think I measure up.

T: Can you think of one or two things you would do differently if you were a better mother?

J (*pause*): Just make a happier home.

T: If a friend told you she wanted to make her home happier, what would you advise her to do?

J: Yell less. And do more things with the kids. Keep things more organized.

T: Are there more things?

J: If I made any of those changes it would be a miracle.

T: OK, let's write a list: "Yell less," "Do more things with the kids," "Keep things more organized." Pick one of the things on this list and let's see if we can get more specific.

J: I don't know which one to pick.

T: Pick one that seems important to you. If they're all important, pick any one you like.

J: Keep things more organized.

T: What would you need to do to get things more organized at home?

J: I don't know. That's my problem.

T: What are the things that let you know you are not organized?

J: I'm late picking up the kids, the house is a mess, I pay my bills late even when I have the money, there're usually dirty dishes in the sink. Do you want more?

T: I get the picture. What would be one or two small changes you could make in the next few weeks that would signal you that your were making progress?

J: I guess if the house was more picked up. And if I was at school when the kids get out.

T: Let's write those two goals over here under "Keep things more organized."

As this session shows, goal setting requires patience and persistence. When Judy has difficulty being specific, the therapist shifts perspective and asks her about a friend. Most clients who become lost in their own experience can think more clearly about someone else. Although it can take time to specify goals in this amount of detail, it is easier to achieve specified goals than vague goals. Also, Judy will see her progress in therapy more clearly if she sets clear, measurable goals.

In this session, Judy and her therapist discuss in detail the changes she needs to make to get her life more organized in the two ways she specified. Clear goals and a plan for achieving them set the stage for Judy either to make desired changes or to discover what thoughts, feelings, and life circumstances interfere with progress in this area of her life.

Constantly Changing Client Goals

A second common difficulty is maintaining focus on set goals. Sometimes it is helpful to change therapy goals. For example, once Betty learned to identify feelings and automatic thoughts, she discovered that she was angry, not depressed. Betty and her therapist shifted their focus to understanding and asserting anger rather than withdrawing, a behavior she and her therapist had misinterpreted as depression. But some clients change therapy goals so often that it is not therapeutic because they don't make progress in any areas of their lives. Observe how Bob's therapist discusses this therapy problem with him.

T: What do you want to make sure we cover today, Bob?

B: I'd like help figuring out how to meet someone to date.

T: Anything else?

B: No. That's the main thing I want help with.

T: Last week we began talking about your plans to change jobs. Should we continue talking about that this week as well?

B: That's not so much on my mind this week.

T: OK. But before we begin talking about dating, I have a concern I'd like to talk over with you, Bob.

B: What's that? Are you upset with me about something?

T: No. Do I seem upset?

B: Not upset exactly. But real serious.

T: I guess I do feel serious because I'm concerned about whether I am helping you as much as I could. Each week you come here with a different problem. Each of these problems is quite upsetting to you, but we don't seem to stick to any one problem long enough to begin to solve it. Have you noticed that?

B: Are you saying you want to get rid of me?

T: Not at all. I want to make sure the therapy is helping you as much as possible. I'm worried that if we keep shifting problems, you'll be in the same spot we started when your 12 weeks of therapy are up. What do you think? Do you think you are making progress?

B: I'm not sure. I like coming here.

T: I'm glad you do. What do you think about my idea of trying to improve how much therapy helps you?

B: Maybe that's a good idea, but I'm not sure how to make it different.

T: One idea I have is to pick one of your problems and talk about it every week, for at least part of the session. What would that be like for you?

B: It might be hard. If I'm charged up about something, I want to go with that.

T: Yes, it might. We could talk about whatever has you "charged up" at the beginning of the session and then switch to talking about our regular problem. How would that be?

B: I'm not sure. Maybe OK. What problem would we work on?

T: That would be up to you. I've made a list of all the problems we've talked about so far. Let's take some time today and decide which one of these areas you'd most like to improve.

Bob's therapist directly expresses concern and describes the possible risks of switching goals each week. However, rather than demanding a single goal focus, the therapist questions Bob to discover what his experience has been in therapy. If Bob had said that a single session was enough to solve each of the problems presented to date, the therapist might have agreed to continue this pattern. But Bob seems to affirm the therapist's perception that there has been little clear therapy progress except for development of a positive therapy relationship.

The therapist then asks Bob if he is willing to try a different approach to therapy and proposes one option. Difficulties Bob might have keeping a single goal focus are identified and a plan for accommodating both Bob's style and the therapist's sense of what will be most helpful is devised. Like all therapeutic shifts, Bob and his therapist will treat this change as a behavioral experiment and evaluate its pros and cons in upcoming therapy sessions. If necessary, Bob and his therapist will collaborate to make additional adjustments to maximize therapy effectiveness.

RECOMMENDED READING

Persons, J. (1989). *Cognitive therapy in practice: A case formulation approach.* New York: W.W. Norton.

4

Using MIND OVER MOOD with Depression

Cognitive Therapy of Depression (Beck et al., 1979) provided therapists with the first detailed cognitive therapy treatment protocol.
Today there are specific cognitive therapy treatment protocols for
almost every diagnosis in the Fourth Edition of the *Diagnostic and
Statistical Manual of Mental Disorders* (DSM-IV: APA, 1994). With
greater specificity in our clinical methods, we are better able to help
many more individuals in brief therapy today than we could 20
years ago. The challenge to therapists is that more knowledge is
required to provide state-of-the-art cognitive therapy today than
was previously necessary. Chapters 4 through 7 of this clinician's
guide show you how to use *Mind Over Mood* in ways that are consistent with current cognitive therapy treatment protocols.

Cognitive therapy has been shown in outcome studies to be an
effective brief treatment for outpatient depression (Dobson, 1989;
Hollon & Najavits, 1988), inpatient depression (Miller, Norman &
Keitner, 1989), panic (Salkovskis & Clark, 1991; Sokol, Beck,
Greenberg, Wright, & Berchick, 1989), generalized anxiety (Butler,

69

Fennell, Robson & Gelder, 1991), and eating disorders (Garner & Bemis, 1982). In addition, it can be useful for the treatment of diverse problems ranging from relationship difficulties (Beck, 1988; Baucom & Epstein, 1990; Dattilio & Padesky, 1990) to schizophrenia (Kingdon & Turkington, 1994) and heroin addiction (Woody et al., 1984)

Outcome is increasingly measured not only by treatment success but by relapse prevention. In the area of relapse prevention, cognitive therapy appears to emerge as a treatment of choice. Compared with medication and other psychotherapies, cognitive therapy has been shown to have lower relapse rates for depression (Blackburn, Eunson & Bishop, 1986; Evans et al., 1992; Hollon, Shelton, & Loosen, 1991; Shea et al., 1990; Thase, 1994).

Effective cognitive therapy involves building skills. Research has demonstrated that depressed clients are less likely to relapse if they are capable of identifying, testing, and altering their automatic thoughts (Neimeyer and Feixas, 1990). *Mind Over Mood* was written in step-by-step fashion to reflect the learning sequence that most clients follow to acquire the skills linked to lower relapse rates.

Basic skills taught in cognitive therapy can help clients overcome a variety of mood, behavior, and relationship problems. *Mind Over Mood* can be used to structure and guide the treatment of clients with a wide variety of presenting problems. The four clients introduced in Chapter 1 of the treatment manual and followed through the remainder of the book represent clients with well-defined and discreet diagnoses and clients with multiple problems, clients treated in both inpatient and outpatient settings, clients in both brief and long-term therapy. Clients with whom you work will probably be able to identify with at least one of the four example clients described in the treatment manual.

Research suggests that the effectiveness of cognitive therapy is contingent on the practitioner being faithful to the cognitive model and cognitive therapy principles (Thase, 1994). *Mind Over Mood* was written, in part, to make it easier for you to adhere to the cognitive model, follow the principles that have been demonstrated to be effective, and help you achieve consistent, effective results.

While the fundamental skills we teach in cognitive therapy are similar across client problems, the order and manner in which the skills are taught vary according to client characteristics, diagnosis, therapy setting, and length of treatment available. The remaining chapters of this guide suggest variations in the use of *Mind Over Mood* for different client populations, diagnoses and therapeutic circumstances. Therapists should be familiar with the principles described in *Cognitive Therapy of Depression* (Beck, Rush, Shaw, & Emery, 1979) and with Chapter 10 of *Mind Over Mood* before devising a treatment plan for depressed clients.

We suggest you ask depressed clients to read the Prologue to *Mind Over Mood* first, followed by Chapter 10. Depressed clients should complete the *Mind Over Mood* Depression Inventory (Worksheet 10.1) or some similar brief measure of depression. A depression inventory is a tool with which to gauge the severity of a client's depression, detail the depression symptoms, and provide a baseline on which to measure improvement. The *Mind Over Mood* Depression Inventory was based in part on symptoms outlined in DSM-IV.

Clients can complete the *Mind Over Mood* Depression Inventory regularly and record and monitor their scores on the graph in Worksheet 10.2. This graph provides visible evidence of improvement or lack of improvement, thus indicating whether therapy is helping or needs to be modified in some way. If the client has difficulty graphing depression scores, you can help by completing the graph in session. Clients who are capable can graph their own scores each week after answering the items of the *Mind Over Mood* Depression Inventory. You or your client can duplicate the inventory reprinted in the Appendix of the treatment manual or use the inventory answer sheet in the Appendix to record client answers each week.

After reading Chapter 10 of *Mind Over Mood* and completing the initial depression inventory, the client can read Chapter 1 (Understanding Your Problems). Chapter 1 provides a framework in which clients begin to understand their difficulties and the interventions that will occur in therapy. The problems the client lists on Worksheet 1.1 can be used as a starting point for developing therapy goals.

Clients experiencing moderate to severe depression initially respond more positively to the activity scheduling described in the last half of Chapter 10 of the treatment manual than to the cognitive interventions described in Chapters 4 through 9. If, in your clinical judgment, the client would initially benefit more from behavioral interventions, be certain the client completes Worksheet 10.4 (Weekly Activity Schedule).

After the client completes the Weekly Activity Schedule, you can ask the client the questions on Worksheet 10.5 to guide learning. Most clients discover that they feel less depressed when they are more active, engaged in pleasurable activities, or actually accomplishing something. In the next session, you and the client might use what you learned from Worksheets 10.4 and 10.5 to plan activities the client can do in the following week to decrease depression.

Most depressed clients will need help from a therapist to plan activities. A Weekly Activity Schedule form can be used to write a plan for the upcoming week. However, the client should be encouraged to substitute preferable activities as they occur to him or her. The activity plan made in the therapy session is a backup plan that provides ideas for activities whenever the depressed person is tempted to simply "do nothing" for long periods of time.

While experimenting with activities to improve mood, the client can begin to read Chapters 2 through 7 in *Mind Over Mood* in sequential order. The pace at which the client proceeds through the treatment manual will depend on level of depression, comprehension, and time available to complete the exercises described. Some clients may complete six chapters in the first two or three weeks of therapy. Other clients may require one or more weeks to complete each chapter. Whatever pace a client sets, be certain to discuss what was learned each week and to review completed exercises.

Almost all depressed clients proceed more slowly through Chapter 6 compared with earlier chapters. Learning to look for evidence that contradicts depressive negative thinking is difficult at first. It is not unusual for clients to spend several weeks mastering the skills described in this chapter. If the number of therapy sessions is limited, it may be preferable to meet less often once the client reaches Chapter 6 than to hurry a client in the acquisition of evidence-collecting skills. The key to depression treatment is learning to identify hot depressive thoughts (Chapter 5) and to look for evidence supporting and contradicting hot thoughts (Chapter 6). By the time clients have mastered these skills and the ability to generate alternative or more balanced thoughts (Chapter 7), they have acquired the primary skills necessary to recover from depression.

Chapter 8 (Experiments and Action Plans) of the treatment manual may be used in therapy for depression whenever it seems useful. For example, if a Thought Record (Chapters 4–7) reveals a problem central to the depression (e.g., the negative thought "I'm a bad parent" is supported by evidence and the client consequently sees himself as inadequate), an Action Plan could be used to begin to solve the problem (help this client become a better parent). Also, depressed persons often predict that activities will not be "fun" or "worthwhile" and use these predictions to support inactivity. A portion of Chapter 8 describes how to use experiments to test these types of beliefs. You can either set these experiments up yourself for the client or use the text of Chapter 8 to guide you and the client in this task.

Most depressed people identify with either Marissa or Ben in *Mind Over Mood*. This identification can be used to encourage depressed clients by showing how Marissa and Ben overcome "stuck" points in therapy by developing new skills. Also, clients can see in the Epilogue that Marissa and Ben did not improve in a purely linear way (Figures E.1 and E.2). In fact, you should inform depressed clients that it is normal to experience fluctuations in depression levels throughout treatment.

Most depressed clients who master the skills taught in Chapters 1 through 8 and 10 learn what they need to know to overcome depression and reduce the likelihood that they will face major depression again. These clients do not need to read the remaining chapters of *Mind Over Mood*, although they may wish to read more about anxiety (Chapter 11) or anger, guilt, and shame (Chapter 12) if these emotions are also prevalent in their lives. You may also wish to recommend that depressed clients complete a *Mind Over Mood* Depression Inventory once a month following completion of therapy to detect increases in depression symptoms over the levels at termination of therapy. A score increase of five points or 30% (whichever is greater) could be used as a cue to reread sections of the treatment manual and complete Thought Records for a few weeks to reduce the risk of relapse. It is important to convey to clients that recurrence of depression is not a sign that treatment has failed but a chance to pinpoint areas of continued or new vulnerability and to use the skills learned to resolve the problems. Subsequent depressions will probably be briefer and less severe if clients apply cognitive therapy skills soon after the depressions appear.

Clients who have experienced chronic or lifelong depression need to use the methods described in Chapter 9 (Assumptions and Core Beliefs) of *Mind Over Mood* after mastering the basic skills taught in Chapters 1 through 8 and 10. Most people with histories of chronic depression have developed core assumptions and beliefs (schemas) that maintain mild to moderate levels of depression even when severe depression lifts. Marissa is the case example of this pattern, and some of her core beliefs are described in Chapter 9. In order to break the depression cycle for similar clients, it is necessary to identify the assumptions and schemas associated with their depression. More detail on how to use Chapter 9 to change core assumptions and schemas is given in Chapter 7 of this guide.

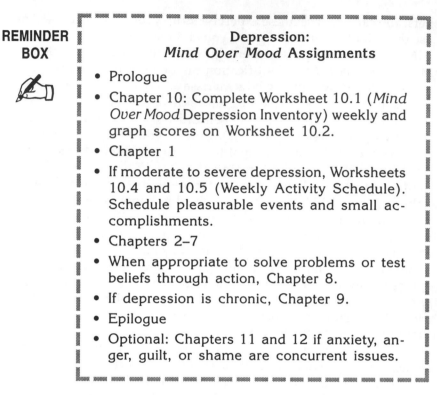

REMINDER BOX

Depression:
Mind Over Mood **Assignments**

- Prologue
- Chapter 10: Complete Worksheet 10.1 (*Mind Over Mood* Depression Inventory) weekly and graph scores on Worksheet 10.2.
- Chapter 1
- If moderate to severe depression, Worksheets 10.4 and 10.5 (Weekly Activity Schedule). Schedule pleasurable events and small accomplishments.
- Chapters 2–7
- When appropriate to solve problems or test beliefs through action, Chapter 8.
- If depression is chronic, Chapter 9.
- Epilogue
- Optional: Chapters 11 and 12 if anxiety, anger, guilt, or shame are concurrent issues.

TROUBLESHOOTING GUIDE

Negativity

One of the hallmarks of depression is negativity. When they begin therapy, many depressed clients are skeptical that *Mind Over Mood* or any other treatment procedure will be helpful. You will lose credibility with a depressed client if you guarantee that therapy will help. Following is a dialogue that has been helpful with depressed clients.

T: (*After presenting the treatment manual and describing its proposed use in therapy*) How does this sound to you? Would you be willing to give this book a try?

C: I don't know. It seems like a lot of work.

T: It will involve some work on your part. Of course, if I could guarantee your work would help you feel better forever, I'm sure you'd give a try. But we can't be sure it will help you. What do you think are the odds it will help?

C: I doubt it will. I've been depressed a long time and nothing helps me.

T: So what's the use of putting out the energy to do this if it won't help, right?

C: Right.

T: I'm glad you let me know you are not very hopeful. Fortunately, if this book is going to help you, it will help even if you don't believe in it. And if it isn't going to help you, we can find that out in just a few weeks of trying it. What do you think about trying this book for a few weeks? Then, based on your experience with the book, we can talk about whether it seems helpful or you or not. If it's not helpful, we can stop using it.

C: Just for two weeks?

T: How about for three weeks? So you give it a fair try.

C: OK. I can do that.

Feeling Overwhelmed

A common experience in depression is feeling overwhelmed. Some depressed clients look at *Mind Over Mood* and want to put it aside because it looks like too much to read and understand. They think worksheets and exercises are too complicated or that they themselves are too stupid or too inept to complete them. When these reactions occur, thank clients for letting you know how they are reacting.

T: When you looked at the Weekly Activity Schedule, your shoulders slumped. What went through your mind?

C: I just can't do this. It's too much.

T: I'm glad to know that's how it seems. Let's see if it is too much. If it is, we can break it into smaller pieces.

C: Maybe I could do a small bit. The whole page just looks too hard.

T: Well, let's try a bit of it together and see how it goes.

C: OK.

T: Right now it's 2:30 on Wednesday. In the 2:00–3:00 P.M. block, what would you write down to describe what you are doing?

C: Counseling.

T: OK. Take this pen and write "Counseling" in that time spot. (*Pauses while client writes.*) Now, how depressed have you been feeling sitting here with me?

C: On this 100-point scale?

T: That's right.

C: About an 80.

T: OK. Write "80" next to the word "Counseling."

(*Therapist and client continue filling out the activity record for earlier hours of the day.*)

T: Well, you've just filled out six hours for today. How long did that take you?

C: I guess about five minutes.

T: Does it seem easier or harder now that you've done part of it?

C: Easier. I guess it's not as hard as I thought.

T: Could you remember back six hours pretty easily?

C: Yes.

T: So maybe you'd need to fill this out only a few times a day. At lunch you could fill it in for the morning, at dinner for the afternoon, and at bedtime for the evening hours.

C: I suppose I could.

T: Let's also talk about how to handle it if you forget to do it one day, or what to do if you get stuck at any point during the week.

As this example shows, depressed clients often feel less overwhelmed when they actually do something than when they think about doing something. It is therefore a good idea to begin all assignments in the therapy session to test beliefs that an assignment will be too difficult. Clients assigned to read a chapter can even practice by reading one paragraph in your office if they are so depressed they think reading will be too difficult.

An additional benefit of beginning therapy assignments in the office is that you can assess whether an assignment is truly too large or difficult for your client. If it is, break it into much smaller pieces or devise a different assignment. If the example client had difficulty remembering activities and rating moods, the therapist might have suggested that the client notice just one time during the week when she felt better and one time when she felt worse and write these down to help her remember them for discussion in the next session.

Hopelessness

A third common element in depression is hopelessness. Hopeless-ness is important to monitor in the treatment of depression because it is a good predictor of suicide. It is critical to reduce hopelessness whenever possible. How do you do this when hopelessness may interfere with client compliance with treatment? One helpful ap-proach is to regularly inquire about hopelessness and acknowledge its credibility to your client. At the same time, it is important to let your client know that you do not find his or her problems hope-less. Further, it can help to provide concrete evidence to your client that expectations of doom do not mean doom is certain. One way to do this is to create hope in response to client negative reactions to *Mind Over Mood* or other aspects of treatment.

T: I notice you completed Worksheet 1-A (Understanding My Prob-lems). What did you learn by doing this?

C: I've got lots of problems. I may as well give up.

T: Let's see. Yes, you do have lots of problems. Would solving even one of these problems help?

C: No. I'd have to solve them all.

T: That's a pretty tough order.

C: So you agree. It's hopeless.

T: Well, if I had to solve them all at once, I'd feel pretty over-whelmed. But I bet if I could solve half of them, the other half would be easier to handle.

C: Maybe. But how could I solve even half of them?

T: Well, you've got me there. That's tough. Whenever I look at more than one problem at once, they seem pretty tough to solve.

C: So you're saying I have to look at one at a time.

T: Well, if we look at one of these problems by itself, I bet we can solve it. If we knock them off one at a time, in a while your life would be much better.

C: How can you fix me getting laid off from my job?

T: Oh, I'm sure we can somehow fix the problems associated with that if we work on them together. But before getting into the de-tails, let's decide if that's the best place to start. First, would you be willing to give my idea a try—to solve one problem at a time?

C: Yeah. For a bit.

T: OK. Let's look at your list here. Why don't you pick which problem we should solve first? Which one do we need to solve to help you most right now?

The therapist simultaneously acknowledges the client's hopelessness and provides an alternative viewpoint. By using guided discovery as described in Chapter 1 of this guide, the therapist helps the client see the advantages of tackling one problem at a time. Making progress in solving one problem will provide more hope to the client than hours of discussion about hope, so it is important to counteract hopelessness with positive problem solving and action. The hopeless client needs to experience some progress and relief from suffering to regain hope. For a thorough discussion of the assessment and treatment of suicidal clients, we recommend *Suicide Risk: Assessment and Response Guidelines* (Fremouw, dePerczel, & Ellis, 1990).

Melancholic Depression

Some depressions are referred to as *melancholic* because they are marked by an almost complete lack of pleasure or responsiveness to positive events. People experiencing this type of depression often have significant physiological symptoms of depression, such as early morning awakening, psychomotor retardation or agitation, and weight loss. These clients can seem as unresponsive to treatment as they are to much of their life experience.

Clients with melancholic depression function at a very low activity level. They may lie in bed or sit in front of the TV for hours with little energy or motivation to do much else. When clients are at such a low level of functioning, therapy should be more behavioral than cognitive. Therapists should focus on the behavioral exercises discussed in Chapter 10 of *Mind Over Mood* and should help energize the depressed client through construction of very small behavioral experiments following the principles outlined in Chapter 8 of the treatment manual. For example, a depressed inpatient who believes "I can't take a walk or do anything but sit in this chair" might be assisted to test this belief in a series of small-step experiments . First, the patient may be helped to stand and walk a few feet from the chair. Following this experiment, the therapist and patient can discuss its meaning.

T: You told me you didn't think you could walk over to the desk. Are you surprised you did it?

P: Yes.

T: What are you feeling right now?

P: Nothing.

T: Do you think you could do it again?

P: I suppose so.

T: I wonder what else you could do if we tried it out?

P: I don't know.

As you can see, the client remains fairly nonresponsive. Notice that the therapist keeps her questions and statements brief and simple to increase the likelihood that the patient will understand what is said. The therapist's questions introduce possibilities that may become meaningful to the client at some point. It is important for the therapist to take a gentle but firm approach in pushing a patient who is this depressed to increase activities in small but meaningful ways. This patient might eventually be encouraged to walk to a day room in the hospital where he will be surrounded by people as he sits.

Melancholic depression, like all severe depressions, is usually treated with a variety of interventions, including medication. When the melancholia lifts, the depressed patient is ready to benefit from cognitive interventions in addition to behavioral experiments.

Discriminating Between Sadness and Depression

People who have experienced recurrent depression or who experience a mixture of grief and depression often have difficulty discriminating between depression and grief or sadness. Some clients think that they need to rid themselves of all sad reactions or they will be susceptible to a return bout of depression. It is helpful to tell clients that sadness and grief are normal, healthy emotions that are part of the human experience. These emotions validate our love for people we have lost and help us learn what we value in life.

One way to teach people to discriminate between sadness or grief and depression is to review the cognitive features of depression described in Chapter 10 of the treatment manual. Thoughts such as "I miss him," "My life is more empty now that she is gone," "I wish this had never happened" signal sadness or grief because they focus on what has been lost. In contrast, depressed thoughts are self-critical ("It's all my fault. I'm no good"), negative about the world ("No one cares for me"), and hopeless about the future ("Things will never get better. Nothing will work out for me"). Sadness and depression often feel similar physiologically and emotionally. The content of our thoughts is often the best way to determine if emotional reactions are healthy grieving or potentially self-destructive depression.

RECOMMENDED READINGS

Beck, A.T., Rush, A.J., Shaw, B.F., & Emery, G. (1979). *Cognitive therapy of depression*. New York: Guilford Press.

Blackburn, I. M., & Davidson, K. (1990). *Cognitive therapy of depression and anxiety*. Oxford: Blackwell.

Freeman, A., & Reinecke, M. (1993). *Cognitive therapy of suicidal behavior*. New York: Springer.

Freemouw, W., de Perczel, M., & Ellis, T. (1990). *Suicide Risk: Assessment and response guidelines*. New York: Pergammon Press.

Gilbert, P. (1994). *Depression: The evolution of powerlessness*. London: LEA.

Scott, J. (1992). Chronic depression: Can cognitive therapy succeed when other treatments fail? *Behavioral & Cognitive Psychotherapy, 20,* 25–36.

Williams, J.M.G. (1992). *The psychological treatment of depression: A general guide to the theory and practice of cognitive behaviour therapy*. London: Routledge.

5

Using MIND OVER MOOD with Anxiety

A specialized cognitive therapy treatment protocol has been designed for each of the anxiety disorders. Therapists have the greatest success in treating anxiety disorders by applying differential treatment approaches to the different types of anxiety. Beck, Emery, and Greenberg (1985) provide a good overview of the cognitive theory of anxiety and a variety of the treatment methods used. More detailed treatment protocols for specific anxiety disorders are provided in Hawton, Salkovskis, Kirk, and Clark (1989). In the following sections, we offer brief guidelines for treating anxiety disorders.

Regardless of the type(s) of anxiety experienced, clients can begin therapy by reading the Prologue of *Mind Over Mood* and then Chapter 11 (Understanding Anxiety). Ask clients to complete the *Mind Over Mood* Anxiety Inventory (Worksheet 11.1) and mark the score on Worksheet 11.2. Clients can complete the anxiety inventory (which assesses the presence of common anxiety symptoms described in DSM-IV) on a weekly basis and record the scores on Worksheet 11.2.

By charting weekly anxiety scores on Worksheet 11.2, clients can observe increases and decreases in anxiety as therapy proceeds. Observing the pattern of change in anxiety scores helps determine when to continue or change the treatment plan. Of course many treatment steps may lead to a temporary increase in anxiety; weekly fluctuations in scores are not as significant as trends sustained over several weeks or more.

For all anxiety disorders it is important that assessment of hot thoughts (*Mind Over Mood*, Chapter 5) includes looking for images. The majority of people who experience anxiety have images when most anxious. Images can be traumatic flashbacks (posttraumatic stress), images of specific feared catastrophic disasters (phobias, generalized anxiety disorder), or repetitive images of violence or sexual acting out (obsessive–compulsive disorder).

GENERALIZED ANXIETY

After reading the Prologue and Chapter 11, clients with generalized anxiety disorder (GAD) can read the rest of *Mind Over Mood* in the sequence written. Some clients may find it useful to complete a Weekly Activity Schedule (*Mind Over Mood*, worksheets 10.4 and 10.5) for one week after reading Chapter 1. In Chapter 10, activity scheduling is described as a stage in depression treatment, but this same worksheet can help therapist and anxious client pinpoint situations or times of the week that particularly trigger anxiety. For example, one client discovered she became most anxious when she had more than one task to do at a time. She later learned to link her anxiety with perfectionistic beliefs. Anxiety triggers can be a focus of intervention in applying skills learned throughout the manual.

Tracking anxious automatic thoughts (*Mind Over Mood*, Chapter 5) helps the person with GAD identify anxious images and "what if?" catastrophic fears. Two types of thinking sustain GAD: overestimations of danger and underestimation of coping ability. Clients can reduce GAD by completing Thought Records (Chapters 5–7): Weighing the evidence diffuses catastrophic certainty, often decreases estimations of danger and increases estimates of coping ability. Chapter 8 is particularly helpful in transforming "what if?" thinking into "then what?" thinking, an important step in increasing clients' confidence in their coping abilities. Chapter 8 can be used to help GAD clients develop coping plans (Action Plans) for each of the foreseen potential disasters. Finally, clients with long-term GAD often have sustaining core beliefs and can benefit from the interventions described in Chapter 9.

REMINDER
BOX

> **Generalized Anxiety: *Mind Over Mood* Assignments**
> - Prologue
> - Chapter 11: Complete Worksheet 11.1 *(Mind Over Mood* Anxiety Inventory) weekly and graph scores on Worksheet 11.2.
> - Chapter 1
> - Worksheet 10.4 (Weekly Activity Schedule). To identify anxiety triggers, Worksheet 10.5.
> - Chapters 2–7 to reevaluate overestimations of danger and underestimations of coping ability.
> - Chapter 8 to transform "what if?" anxious thinking into "then what?" problem solving.
> - If generalized anxiety is chronic, Chapter 9.
> - Epilogue
> - Optional: Chapters 10 and 12 if depression, anger, guilt, or shame are concurrent issues.

PANIC DISORDER

A very specific and highly successful treatment protocol for panic disorder has been developed by Clark (1989). This treatment approach is effective with 80% to 95% of clients within 5 to 20 sessions with less than 10% relapse after one year's follow-up (Clark et al., 1994). A similar treatment has been developed by Barlow (1988). For a more detailed explanation of the cognitive treatment of panic disorder, see Clark (1989).

Multiple lines of research support the cognitive theory of panic, which states that panic disorder results from the catastrophic misinterpretation of internal sensations (physical or mental). People who panic enter a vicious cycle in which sensations are followed by catastrophic beliefs that lead to anxiety and therefore more sensations, as shown in Figure 5.1. Further, people with panic disorder usually avoid activities or experiences associated with feared sensations. For example, a woman who believed a rapid heart rate

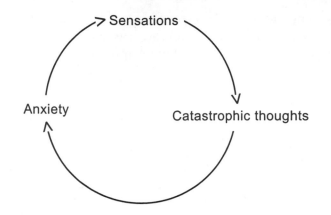

Figure 5.1. Vicious circle in panic disorder.

signaled an oncoming heart attack avoided walking up stairs because this exercise caused her heart rate to increase.

Cognitive therapy of panic disorder involves (1) identifying the catastrophic fears (hot thoughts) linked to sensations (*Mind Over Mood* Chapter 5), (2) inducing sensations to demonstrate the vicious cycle, test catastrophic fears, and identify alternative noncatastrophic explanations for sensations (Chapter 6–8), (3) ongoing behavioral experiments to see whether the catastrophic or noncatastrophic explanations provide a better understanding of the occurrence of sensations (Chapter 8), and (4) behavioral experiments to decrease avoidance behaviors so that clients can discover that feared catastrophes won't happen even under the worst of circumstances (Chapter 8).

To illustrate point 4, one man avoided becoming overheated because he feared that sweating indicated an oncoming heart attack. He did experiments in which he allowed himself to become overheated: He wore sweaters and an overcoat in a warm room to induce sweating beyond normal experience. His catastrophic fear dissipated when he discovered that intense sweating did not bring on a heart attack. In *Mind Over Mood*, Linda is the example client with panic disorder. Chapter 8 of the treatment manual includes a description of the behavioral experiment procedures Linda followed in her therapy to test her catastrophic fears and reduce avoidance behaviors.

A common therapist error is using cognitive therapy for panic disorder with clients who experience panic attacks but do not have panic disorder. Clients with any type of severe anxiety can experience panic attacks. The panic treatment described here should be applied only when panic attacks are not symptomatic of another anxiety diagnosis; that is, when at least some panic attacks occur "spontaneously" rather than in response to a feared situation.

REMINDER BOX

> **Panic Disorder:** *Mind Over Mood* **Assignments**
> * Prologue
> * Chapter 11: Complete Worksheet 11.1 (*Mind Over Mood* Anxiety Inventory) weekly and graph scores on Worksheet 11.2.
> * Chapters 4–7, with particular attention to Linda's descriptions of her panic, to identify and test catastrophic fears and alternative, noncatastrophic explanations for sensations.
> * Chapter 8 to guide behavioral experiments in which sensations are induced to (a) test catastrophic explanations of sensations, (b) weigh the evidence supporting catastrophic and noncatastrophic explanations for sensations, and (c) improve client confidence that catastrophes won't happen as client decreases avoidance behaviors.
> * Epilogue
> * Optional: Other chapters that are of interest to the client or that teach skills the client is lacking.

Because the treatment of panic disorder is very specific clients who are in treatment for panic disorder alone need to read only a few chapters of *Mind Over Mood.* A brief case description illustrates this abbreviated treatment model.

In session 1, the therapist assesses Roger, a 46-year-old welder, and determines that he meets criteria for panic disorder. The therapist asks Roger to read the Prologue and Chapter 11 of *Mind Over Mood* and to complete the *Mind Over Mood* Anxiety Inventory before the next session.

In session 2, the therapist interviews Roger about a severe panic attack he had the previous week, using the questions that help identify hot thoughts in the Helpful Hints box on page 51. The questioning follows that suggested by Clark (1989) and quickly pinpoints the catastrophic fear related to sensations.

T: When your panic was at its worst, what sensations did you experience?

R: I couldn't get my breath. My heart was pounding.

T: Anything else?

R: I was hot and sweaty. I felt as if I would pass out.

T: Anything else?

R: No.

T: And when you couldn't get your breath, your heart was pounding, you felt hot and sweaty, and felt as if you would pass out, what went through your mind?

R: I don't know. My head was swimming.

T: What was the worst thing you imagined might happen?

R: I thought I was having a heart attack.

T: Did you have any images of yourself having a heart attack?

R: Yes, I did. I saw myself on the ground and I was white and my eyes were closed and the paramedics were coming.

T: In this image, what had happened?

R: I had a heart attack. And I thought I was dead.

T: And when you had that image, how did that make you feel?

R: Scared.

T: How do you think that scared feeling affected your breathing, heart rate, and sweating?

R (pauses): Well, when I'm scared, I guess my heart beats faster and sometimes I sweat more then. I'm not sure about my breathing.

T: Those are interesting observations. We'll have to pay attention to your breathing when you get scared and see what we can learn about that. For now, let's draw a picture of what we have discovered about your panic so far (draws a diagram similar to Figure 5.1, using the client's owns words and reported experiences).

By the end of the second session, Roger has a clearer idea of the link between his physical sensations, his catastrophic thoughts about these sensations ("I'm having a heart attack," an image of lying dead on the floor), and panic. The therapist suggests that Roger read Chapters 5 and 6 of *Mind*

Over Mood, paying particular attention to how Linda in Chapter 6 looks for evidence to support her fear that she is having a heart attack.

In session 3, Roger and his therapist induce the sensations that frighten Roger to look for alternative explanations for them. (Note: All clients presenting with symptoms of anxiety should have a medical clearance that rules out physical illness. Roger had been examined by his general physician and a cardiologist, neither of whom found evidence of a heart problem.) Sensations are induced by running in place, hyperventilating, and imagining his most recent panic attack. These inductions (chosen for their similarity to Roger's panic experiences) lead Roger to conclude that exercise, changes in breathing, and anxious mental imagery can all bring on the sensations he assumed were indicators of a heart attack.

By the end of this session, Roger is only 50% certain that breathlessness, a racing heart, sweating, and lightheadedness are dangerous. The therapist asks Roger to read Chapter 7 of *Mind Over Mood* and compare his experiences in the third session with Linda's panic experiences as described in the manual. During the coming week Roger also tries to discover alternative, noncatastrophic explanations for troubling sensations that occur.

In session 4, Roger and his therapist continue to induce sensations and discuss noncatastrophic explanations for sensations that occurred "spontaneously" during the week. Roger reports a steady decline in his scores on the *Mind Over Mood* Anxiety Inventory and a decrease in panic attacks from daily to only two times in the preceding week. The therapist helps Roger devise a series of experiments he can do in the coming week to continue to evaluate whether his catastrophic or non-catastrophic explanations best explain his physical sensations. His reading assignment is Chapter 8 of *Mind Over Mood*, in which Linda does her own experiments.

In the next three sessions, Roger and his therapist continue to review and evaluate his experiments inside and outside the office. They identify a few avoidance behaviors that Roger uses for "safety" and "heart attack prevention," such as reducing his workout at the gym. Roger conducts experiments in which he violates his safety rules to see if he can bring on a heart attack through exercise.

By the end of therapy, Roger feels 100% certain that his sensations are not catastrophic and can be explained by changes in breathing or anxiety or ingestion of caffeine. He has not experienced panic attack for two weeks. The therapist advises Roger to bring on the sensations at least once a week in the upcoming months to bolster his confidence that they are not dangerous. He can also review the treatment steps in *Mind Over Mood* if necessary.

PHOBIAS

Clients with phobias can use *Mind Over Mood* to help identify the hot thoughts that accompany their fear (Chapter 5). One of the best questions to identify a hot thought for anxiety is "What is the worst thing that could happen?" The therapist asks this question over and over again to uncover layers of fears and teaches clients to ask themselves the question.

Thought Records (*Mind Over Mood*, Chapters 4–7) can help evaluate fears. An important step in overcoming phobias is to develop coping plans for managing the feared situation. Once a coping plan has been developed, phobic avoidance can be overcome through experiments and Action Plans (Chapter 8) to evaluate the effectiveness of the coping plan. With phobias, experiments and Action Plans are usually done in hierarchical fashion, as described in Chapter 11 of *Mind Over Mood*.

It is critically important for clients with phobias to approach and cope with their fears either in actuality or, if necessary, in imagery. For example, fear of a plane crash can be confronted in imagery. The client who fears a plane crash can develop coping plans to increase their survival chances and also to prepare for death in the case of not surviving a crash. Coping training often helps a client who is not reassured by the low probability of a crash. Chapter 8 worksheets are helpful in developing coping plans.

It is very important that hot thoughts remain a focus of therapy. Thus, clients with social phobia who fear rejection should be exposed to rejection and be taught to cope with it. Exposure exercises often can be done in the therapy hour through role-play with the therapist. Socially phobic clients can learn in role-plays to assertively defend themselves against criticism, as shown in the following example.

C: I just can't go to that meeting. I'll be too anxious.

T: What is the worst thing that might happen if you go?

C: They'll see what a poor job I'm doing.

T: Let's make a list of all the negative things they might think of you, and then we can prepare a plan to cope with criticisms if they occur.

(Client lists seven different feared criticisms over the next five minutes of discussion.)

T: Now let's take each of these criticisms and see how you could respond if someone at the meeting actually said this or thought this about you. Which one would you like to start with?

C: "You're stupid."

T: OK. I seem to recall that that thought came up on one of your Thought Records this week.

C: Yes, right here (points to Worksheet 6.1).

T: Why don't you read aloud the evidence you came up with that did not support this thought.

C (reading): I graduated from high school. The other mechanics think I have good ideas when we're talking in the cafeteria one-on-one. I know how to make lots of things in my garage.

T: When you read that list, do you feel stupid?

C: No. I just feel stupid when I'm in a big group and get tongue-tied.

T: Try saying this: "I'm not stupid. I just get tongue-tied in groups. One-on-one I can explain my ideas better."

C: I'm not stupid. I just get tongue-tied in groups. One-on-one I can explain my ideas better.

T: How do you feel when you say that?

C: Better. It's true.

T: Let's come up with a response that seems true to you and makes you feel better for the other six criticisms, and then we can practice saying or thinking these statements when you think others are criticizing you.

Agoraphobia can be treated with these same guidelines: identify the fears (Chapter 5), evaluate the danger (Chapters 6–7), and develop coping plans, approaching what has been avoided in a hierarchical fashion (Chapter 8). If the client experiences panic with agoraphobia, the panic treatment is usually treated first, agoraphobic avoidance second. Sometimes family or couples therapy is necessary to help identify beliefs (Chapters 5 and 9) in the family system that support agoraphobia. Family members can use Thought Records and behavioral experiments in *Mind Over Mood* (Chapters 6–8) to help evaluate their own beliefs that interfere with the agoraphobic family member's progress.

REMINDER BOX

> **Phobias: *Mind Over Mood* Assignments**
> - Prologue
> - Chapter 11: Complete Worksheet 11.1 (*Mind Over Mood* Anxiety Inventory) weekly and graph scores on Worksheet 11.2.
> - Chapters 4–7 to uncover hot thoughts ("What's the worst that could happen?").
> - Chapter 8 to develop coping plans for fears; practice these coping plans using a fear hierarchy (described in Chapter 11).
> - Epilogue
> - Optional: Other chapters that are of interest to the client or that teach skills the client is lacking.

OBSESSIVE–COMPULSIVE DISORDER

Gail Steketee has written very informative books on the treatment of obsessive–compulsive disorder (OCD) for both therapists (1993) and clients (1990). Since treatment of OCD can be quite complex, therapists are urged to read these or similar texts before attempting to treat OCD for the first time. Once you are familiar with the cognitive–behavioral treatment for OCD (see also Salkovskis, 1988, 1989), *Mind Over Mood* can be a helpful adjunct. For example, completion of a Weekly Activity Schedule (Worksheet 10.4) can help you and the client identify precipitants of either obsessional thinking or compulsive behavior.

While the standard behavioral treatment for OCD involves exposure (e.g., to dirt for a client with fear of contamination) and response prevention (e.g., no hand washing following exposure to dirt), what the client should do during the response prevention period is not defined. Response prevention should last until the exposure anxiety dissipates, which can take minutes or hours. Cognitive interventions can be used to help clients comply with the response prevention directive. During this time the client can identify and test OCD-related thoughts, such as "The anxiety will never go away if I can't wash."

REMINDER BOX

> ## Obsessive–Compulsive Disorder:
> ### *Mind Over Mood* Assignments
> - Prologue
> - Chapter 11: Complete Worksheet 11.1 (*Mind Over Mood* Anxiety Inventory) weekly and graph scores on Worksheet 11.2.
> - Worksheet 10.4 (Weekly Activity Schedule). Worksheet 10.5 to identify anxiety triggers.
> - Chapter 12, especially the section on guilt, to help reduce some types of OCD thinking. For example, the Responsibility Pie (Worksheet 12.2) technique can be used to assess responsibility fears.
> - Chapter 8 to develop a coping plan for disasters that could occur so that disasters do not need to be "prevented" by compulsions; to construct experiments to test OCD-related thoughts.
> - Chapters 4–7. Caution: do not test OCD thoughts themselves, such as "This will make my children ill." Instead, test beliefs about OCD, such as "Thinking something means it will happen."
> - Optional: Other chapters that are of interest to the client or that teach skills the client is lacking.

There is no empirical data thus far to suggest that using Thought Records to test OCD thoughts (e.g., "Touching a doorknob will give me cancer") improves treatment outcome. However, Salkovskis and his colleagues (Salkovskis, 1988; Salkovskis 1989; Salkovskis & Kirk, 1989) are evaluating a cognitive treatment model in which therapist and client test beliefs regarding responsibility (e.g., "If my mother gets ill, it's my fault") and the meaning of OCD thoughts. For example, therapist and client can use Thought Records to test beliefs such as "Having OCD thoughts means I'm a bad person," or "Thinking this will make it happen (or is as bad as wanting it to happen)". Early research data suggest that these types of cognitive interventions which target the meaning of OCD thoughts may improve treatment outcome.

POSTTRAUMATIC STRESS DISORDER AND ACUTE STRESS DISORDER

Clients who seek therapy following a trauma can use *Mind Over Mood* to build skills to cope with trauma's aftermath. However, treatment of postraumatic stress disorder involves much more than learning to cope, so *Mind Over Mood* can be only a segment of the treatment. Therapists working with trauma survivors can learn more about trauma treatment by reading recent books describing cognitive therapy approaches to trauma (Foy, 1992; Meichenbaum, 1994; Resick & Schnicke, 1993; Saigh, 1992).

Use of *Mind Over Mood* depends on the type (single incident or chronic) and recency of trauma. Generally, recent trauma, especially if a single incident (e.g., earthquake, robbery, fire), is treated with critical incident stress debriefing, as described by Mitchell (1983). Clients experiencing recent trauma can use *Mind Over Mood* to better understand the link between the trauma and current experiences (Chapter 1), help identify feelings (Chapter 3), identify thoughts (Chapter 5), and develop coping plans (Chapter 8) for trauma recovery.

People who experience chronic or severe traumas may develop core survival beliefs that are maladaptive in nontrauma circumstances (e.g., "No one can be trusted"). These core beliefs can be evaluated using the methods described in Chapter 9 of the treatment manual. It is helpful for trauma survivors to learn when to use protective beliefs and when it is safe to employ alternative beliefs. Also, the methods used for overcoming guilt and shame described in Chapter 12 are helpful for some trauma survivors.

Regardless of the type or number of traumas a person has survived, an important part of recovery is learning to discover constructive personal meaning in the trauma and apply it to one's view of oneself, others, and the world. *Mind Over Mood* teaches skills that can facilitate this process for many people.

REMINDER BOX

Posttraumatic Stress Disorder:
Mind Over Mood **Assignments**

- Prologue
- Chapter 11: Complete Worksheet 11.1 (*Mind Over Mood* Anxiety Inventory) weekly and graph scores on Worksheet 11.2.
- Chapter 1
- Worksheet 10.4 (Weekly Activity Schedule). Worksheet 10.5 identify PTSD triggers.
- Chapter 3 to help identify and discriminate among emotional reactions.
- Chapter 5 to identify hot thoughts and images maintaining PTSD.
- Chapters 6 and 7 to look for additional personal meaning in trauma.
- Chapter 8 to develop coping plans for potential future traumas.
- Chapter 9 to evaluate core beliefs that are not currently adaptive.
- Optional: Chapters 10 and 12 if depression, anger, guilt or shame are concurrent issues.

TROUBLESHOOTING GUIDE

Difficulty Identifying Anxious Thoughts

Anxious clients sometimes cannot identify the content of their thoughts when anxious. For example, when you ask, "What was going through your mind just before you anxiously fled the shopping mall?" an anxious client might reply, "I don't know. I just felt really bad and had to get out of there." There are several ways to help the anxious client identify thoughts when they seem inaccessible. Use of imagery is often the key.

When anxious, we avoid. Avoidance is often cognitive as well as behavioral; many anxious thoughts are pushed out of the mind as soon as they occur. Therefore, clients literally have trouble accessing thoughts that may be key to understanding their anxiety. One way to deal with avoidance is to bring the anxiety into the present in the office and stay alert to even momentary, fleeting thoughts that accompany or precede anxiety. Using imagery, most clients can reexperience any anxiety-related event, as in the following example.

T: What was going through your mind just before you anxiously fled the shopping mall?

C: I don't know. I just felt really bad and had to get out of there.

T: Let's see if we can recapture your thoughts by returning to the shopping mall right now. I'd like you to imagine yourself at the shopping mall just as it was yesterday. Take a few minutes and see if you can vividly recall the scene—sights, sounds, smells, and what you were feeling inside.

C: (*Pauses*) OK.

T: Describe to me what is going on.

C: I'm holding a heavy shopping bag and my daughter is tugging on my arm. There are people rushing everywhere and I can't decide where I need to go next.

T: What are you feeling?

C: I'm hot and my mind seems all confused. I can't quite figure out where I am. All the stores look strange to me.

T: What's going through your mind?

C: I don't know. My mind seems odd. I think I'm losing it.

T: You think you're losing your mind?

C: Yes. I feel like I'm going crazy. Who will take care of my daughter?

T: Do you have any mental pictures of this?

C: I see my mother with her hair all tangled and her eyes wild like she got when she was drunk when I was a kid. I think I look like that to my daughter.

T: How does that image make you feel?

C: (*Breathes rapidly*) Very anxious. I've got to stop now. (Opens eyes in fear.)

T: How similar was your experience today to what you felt yesterday?

C: That's exactly how I felt. I had forgotten about that picture of my mother. I do get scared that I look like that to my daughter.

This session excerpt illustrates how imagery can help a client recapture anxious feelings and the accompanying thoughts during the therapy session. It is important to help the client experience anxiety within the therapy hour in order to identify and test anxious thoughts, as well as to evaluate the helpfulness of different therapeutic interventions. This example also highlights the importance of asking about images when the client is anxious. In this illustration, the client has a thought, "I'm going crazy," that helps explain her anxiety. However, the image of her mother with wild eyes and tangled hair proves to be a much more vivid trigger for her anxiety.

Chapter 5 of *Mind Over Mood* reminds all clients to look for images and memories and to list them in the "Automatic Thoughts" column of the Thought Record when trying to understand a mood. This point should be emphasized for anxious clients, most of whom have images during peak anxiety. When testing automatic thoughts (*Mind Over Mood* Chapter 6), it is important to evaluate these images as well as word thoughts. For example, the particular client in the case excerpt might be given a mirror in session when she becomes highly anxious and has an image of herself as a crazy woman. She can compare her image in the mirror with the image in her mind. She could also benefit from comparing her internal experience to insanity to develop confidence that she is not going crazy when anxious. Finally, her emotional and cognitive reactions to her drunken mother when she was a child should be explored and related to her fears of her adult emotional responses.

Desire to Eliminate Anxiety

Anxious clients often want to set a therapy goal to eliminate anxiety. This goal is not therapeutic because it implies that it is desirable (and possible) to avoid all anxiety. Also, a client who wants to eliminate anxiety will often balk at necessary therapeutic interventions that lead to a temporary increase in anxiety. Further, since it is impossible to eliminate anxiety, a client who maintains this goal will view therapy as a failure when anxiety reappears. The belief that anxiety is "bad" should therefore be identified and evaluated early in therapy:

T: What is your goal for our therapy?
C: I want to get rid of my anxiety.

T: Totally?

C: Yes.

T: Well, I need to tell you right away that I can't help you do that. And even if I could, I don't think it would be a good idea.

C: What do you mean?

T: Let's see how I can explain this. (Pauses.) Do you have a smoke alarm in your house?

C: Yes.

T: Has it ever gone off when there was no fire?

C: Sure. When I'm cooking the oven sometimes smokes.

T: Sometimes I cook by smoke alarm—when the alarm goes off, dinner is done. (Both laugh.) But as annoying as it is when the alarm blasts when there's no real fire, do you think it would be a good idea to permanently disconnect the alarm?

C: No.

T: Why not?

C: Because you want the alarm there for when there is a real fire.

T: Yes. And that's why I don't think it's a good idea to get rid of your anxiety.

C: You mean my anxiety is like a smoke alarm?

T: Uh huh. Anxiety is your body's signal that there might be danger. Now, most of the time there is no danger, but sometimes there is, so you want to keep your alarm in place.

C: Then I'm stuck with feeling anxious?

T: Sometimes. But what we can do in therapy is help you learn to tell more quickly if there is real danger and how to turn the alarm off sooner if there's no danger. This way you'll feel anxious less often and for shorter amounts of time. But your anxiety will still be there when you need it.

C: OK. I guess that would be an improvement.

T: Our first goal, then, will be to learn what is causing your anxiety alarm to go off. Instead of trying to stop your anxiety this week, would you be willing to observe carefully when it happens and try to figure out what is causing it to go off?

C: What should I look for?

T: When you get anxious, try to notice what is going on around you, what you are feeling, and what thoughts go through your mind just before your alarm goes off. The treatment manual has a worksheet, Worksheet 5.3), called a Thought Record, that you can use to record your observations. Try to fill out the first three columns of this worksheet two or three times this week when you feel anxious to help us learn what sorts of things set off your anxiety alarm. Chapter 5 teaches you how to do this.

C: OK, I'll give that a try.

The therapist in this example uses a metaphor to teach the client that anxiety can be beneficial. Further, she encourages the client to adopt a curious attitude toward anxiety rather than an antagonistic attitude. It is important for anxious clients to become observers of their anxiety rather than avoiders of anxiety. Only by observing, understanding, and facing anxiety do people learn to cope with it better.

Avoidance of Therapy Procedures

Since avoidance is a hallmark of anxiety, it is not surprising that anxious clients often want to avoid therapy procedures, especially since the procedures often lead to a temporary increase in anxiety. Clients may say they don't want to recall images, approach feared situations, or even write down their anxious thoughts on a Thought Record. It is our role as therapists to shepherd clients through these experiences without creating an antagonistic struggle. If we take small steps, teach coping skills, and adeptly test anxious beliefs, anxious clients can overcome avoidance.

T: Since you had trouble figuring out what was going through your mind when you were anxious this week, let me help you get anxious in the session today and maybe we can figure out the thoughts together.

C: No, I don't want to do that today.

T: Why not?

C: I'm not having a good day. I don't think I'd handle getting anxious very well.

T: What do you think would happen?

C: I'd probably start shaking all over and couldn't stop.

T: Do you have a mental picture of yourself doing that?

C: Yes. (*Shakes head.*) I don't want to think about it.

T: Well, we have a bit of a dilemma, then. You see, in order for me to help you learn to handle your anxiety, we need to have you experience it.

C: I know. But let's do it another day.

T: That would be one approach. Although, if you're already feeling bad today, this might be a good day to start.

C: Yes. But I know I can't handle it.

T: Would you be willing to take a tiny, tiny step to test that idea?

C: What do you mean?

T: Well, for example, do you think you could handle thinking about what makes you anxious for about 30 seconds? After 30 seconds I'll help you reduce your anxiety. We can talk about other things or do relaxation or do whatever it takes to help you feel better. Do you think you would start shaking uncontrollably after 30 seconds?

C: I might. I'm not sure.

T: Would you be willing to try? I absolutely promise to help you feel less anxious after that time period.

C: All right.

T: Just think about what happened on Friday, then, when you felt so anxious. Let your mind recall it really clearly for 30 seconds. I'll watch the time and interrupt you after 30 seconds.

(*Client closes eyes and imagines for 30 seconds.*)

T: Stop! OK, let's talk about television for a bit. Do you have a favorite show? Tell me about it.

(*Client talks to therapist for a few minutes about a favorite television episode.*)

T: Let's stop this for awhile. How are you feeling right now?

C: Pretty good. Not too anxious.

T: How did you feel after 30 seconds of thinking about Friday?

C: I was starting to get anxious.

T: How close were you to shaking uncontrollably?

C: I guess not very close.

T: So do you think our plan worked okay? Were you able to feel anxious and then feel better again?

C: Yes, it was better than I expected.

T: Maybe we can help you with your anxiety in small steps like this. For instance, we could try 60 seconds of thinking about what makes you anxious and then help you calm down. If that goes all right, we could try two minutes. In two minutes we could probably learn some important information about your anxiety without you taking too big a risk. What do you think?

C: I would try a little bit more. As long as I can signal if I want to stop.

T: That's a deal. We can do a lot of small experiments with brief anxiety until you become more confident. Of course, eventually we'll want to test the idea that you will shake uncontrollably if you really let your anxiety loose, but we can increase your confidence in handling small and medium amounts of anxiety before we tackle that.

C: You really think this is necessary for me to feel better?

T: I really do. Ready to try one minute?

C: I guess so, if you think it will help.

Notice how the therapist gently pushes the anxious client to test her belief that she will shake uncontrollably if exposed to anxious thoughts. It is important for the therapist to balance respect for the client's fear with the knowledge that avoidance only fuels anxiety. It is much better to take small steps forward in anxiety treatment than to stop progress because a client is unwilling to take a bigger step.

Reliance on Medication

Some of the dangers of long-term medication treatment of anxiety problems are discussed in Chapter 11 of *Mind Over Mood*. The most serious problems arise with long-term use of tranquilizers, which can lead to addiction, tolerance effects, and rebound anxiety when medication is withdrawn. However, reliance on any type of medication that dampens the anxiety response can lead to interference with the practice of psychotherapeutic methods of anxiety management. Therefore, it is usually desirable to work with the prescribing physician to help the anxious client taper off medication as soon as possible after psychotherapeutic treatment begins. The exception to this recommendation is in the treatment of clients who experience anxiety so debilitating that it is difficult for them to participate in therapy. These clients often benefit from short-term use of medication until they have learned skills to manage anxiety unassisted.

Some clients balk at the idea of reducing medication, even if the prescribing physician and the therapist agree that it is safe and desirable to do so. Others don't mind reducing medication but are unwilling to stop taking it completely, clinging to a tiny partial dose as insurance against the return of full-blown anxiety. Client beliefs in the necessity of medication are important to test because the beliefs are usually rooted in a conviction that anxiety itself is dangerous and uncontrollable and that the blocking response of medication is required because other treatments are ineffective. These beliefs, if untested, can undermine the client's motivation to practice and rely on skills learned in therapy.

To shift beliefs about medication, it is usually necessary to combine information with behavioral experiments. It is helpful if the client's physician corroborates the therapist's information about the safety of managing anxiety without medication. If the physician believes that pharmacological treatment is necessary for anxiety, the therapist must propose similar information and behavioral experiments to the physician.

The following excerpt illustrates how didactic information can be conveyed via guided discovery. Guided discovery reduces the likelihood that the client will respond "Yes, but . . . " to information related to the reduction of medication.

T: You have been unwilling to experiment with going into a meeting without taking a small dose of Xanax. I'd like to discuss that decision today.

C: I know you don't want me to take the medication. But I don't think it hurts anything and it helps me not avoid the meetings, like I used to.

T: That's the advantage of the medication. Can you think of any disadvantages?

C: No.

T: What do you think would happen if you didn't take the medication?

C: I'd probably get panicky and leave the meeting.

T: What would be an alternative to leaving if you became panicky?

C: Well, I suppose I could try practicing relaxation, and I could also identify and test my thoughts.

T: How confident are you that these strategies would work as well as the medication?

C: If I'm honest with you, not very confident.

T: That's what I thought. What would it take for you to become confident?

C: I guess I'd have to try them out without medication and see if they work. But it's just too risky to try that at a meeting where I could make a fool of myself in front of customers.

T: Suppose you had a friend whom you wanted to encourage to get off medication. What would you advise him in this situation?

C: (*Smiling*) You're tricking me.

T: I don't mean to trick you. It just seems that you can think of only one way to handle this for yourself. I thought maybe you could get more ideas if we shifted the focus off you.

C: Well, I might tell my friend to try not taking the medication before a meeting that is less pressured. In some meetings I don't have to say much. Or I could take the medication with me and only take it if my anxiety gets bad and the other techniques don't work.

T: Those are two good ideas you could try out. How long would it take the medication to work if you did take it as a last-minute backup?

C: Usually I feel better within a few minutes.

T: Really?

C: You seem surprised.

T: I am. Xanax usually takes at least 15 or 20 minutes to take effect. Do you really feel better within a few minutes of taking it?

C: Yes, I do.

T: Then how would you explain that? Why do you think you feel calmer in a few minutes if the medication takes 15 to 20 minutes to have a physiological effect?

C: Maybe because I feel reassured that help is on the way.

T: So your confidence in the Xanax might help you even before the medication does?

C: Yes, that makes sense.

T: Does it also make sense then that increasing your confidence in relaxation and the cognitive methods you've been learning in *Mind Over Mood* might help make these methods more helpful, too?

C: Yes, I think it would.

T: Perhaps it's time to do some experiments to find out if you can be as confident in these other methods as you are in the medication. Which experiment would you be willing to try first?

C: Maybe to not take the medication at a less pressured meeting, but to still carry the medication with me in case my anxiety gets too bad.

T: That seems like a good place to start. Let's review what you'll do instead of taking medication. Also, we should make some backup plans so you don't take the medication at the slightest hint of anxiety.

C: (*Laughs*) Yes, I might want to do that!

It often takes a number of weeks to convince a client who firmly believes in medication that other methods can be as effective. Therefore, it is a good idea to identify beliefs about medication early in therapy so you can devise experiments to test them as soon as the client learns other anxiety management strategies. Clients who have been on medication long enough to experience withdrawal effects when the medication is reduced should be warned of the probability of temporarily increased anxiety. Withdrawal anxiety can be reframed as an opportunity to try out cognitive and relaxation strategies for reducing anxiety when the cause of the anxiety (in this case, physiological withdrawal) cannot be changed.

Mixed Anxiety Problems

Many anxious clients enter therapy with a mix of anxiety problems. One client may experience panic as well as social anxiety. Another may have a long history of generalized anxiety yet enter therapy for help with a phobia. How do you know what treatment protocol to follow? One strategy is to define the different problems and ask the client which one he or she would like to tackle first. Very often, however, all anxiety problems are equally important to the client. In this case, it is helpful to see if there is a central theme that links the anxiety problems and/or the treatment protocols. Identification of overlapping themes or treatment skills needed often leads to an individualized treatment plan that meets all the client's anxiety needs, as illustrated in the following case example.

Monique entered therapy with generalized anxiety compounded by a social phobia and recent onset of panic attacks. In the first session, Monique described herself as a perfectionist. Her father had been very punitive when she was a child, and she had struggled to do things perfectly to avoid his criticism and punishment. Throughout her life Monique experienced intense anxiety whenever she was in a large social situation and could not be sure that everyone in the room approved of her.

Monique's anxiety intensified after she moved to a new city. She was afraid that her new neighbors and other people would notice her anxiety and think she was crazy. These thoughts were followed by increased anxiety and depersonalization experiences that Monique interpreted as evidence that she was in fact going crazy. Each time she thought she was going crazy she experienced a panic attack. Monique described herself as "caught in a storm" of anxiety.

Although Monique was experiencing three problems—generalized anxiety, panic, and social phobia—all three stemmed from her fear of criticism. The therapist therefore decided to help Monique learn to cope with criticism better so that it didn't frighten her so much. The first week the therapist suggested that Monique read the Prologue and Chapter 11 of *Mind Over Mood*. In addition, he asked her to complete a Weekly Activity Schedule (Worksheet 10.4) to discover the pattern in her anxiety for herself.

After observing that many social situations greatly increased her anxiety, Monique learned to identify her thoughts in these situations using the guidelines in Chapter 5 of the treatment manual. These thoughts focused on the fear and certainty that others were critical of her and would punish her in some way. Using the strategies in Chapter 8, Monique and her therapist developed assertion Action Plans that she could put into effect if other people criticized her. For example, she role-played defending her anxiety to a stranger who acted in accordance with her worst-case scenario.

T: (*Roleplaying a critical stranger*) You look like you're going crazy.

M: Actually, I'm just feeling anxious right now.

T: Well, it seems pretty crazy to me to be anxious just walking down the street.

M: Maybe you don't feel anxious here. Different people feel anxious in different situations.

T: You look odd. I think maybe I should call an ambulance.

M: Just leave me alone. I'm OK. I'll feel better if you leave.

T: I don't like how you look. You stay here and I'll call 911.

M: You have no right to meddle in someone else's life. Just go away!

In role-play exercises such as this, Monique learned to speak up for herself, defending her anxiety or any other aspect of her behavior that others might criticize. She was surprised that, after repeated role-plays, she became angry with criticism and could see that it was generally unwarranted in the situations in which she feared it. By developing Action Plans to cope with the possibility of criticism, her anxiety decreased in social situations. She also became less fearful of strangers and experienced depersonalization less often. Defending her anxiety led Monique to become confident that she was not going crazy, and her panic also subsided. By pinpointing the central theme connecting all her anxiety problems, Monique and her therapist were able to help her overcome most of her anxiety in a few months using the skills taught in *Mind Over Mood*.

The table on the following page shows the types of cognitions associated with the most common anxiety problems. A brief summary of the primary treatment interventions used to help these problems is also provided along with a list of the treatment manual chapters that teach relevant skills.

Anxiety, Cognitions, Interventions, and *Mind Over Mood* Assignments

Anxiety type	Common cognitions	Interventions	Mind Over Mood assignments
Generalized anxiety	What if? Overestimate danger Underestimate coping Vulnerability schemas	Identify triggers Look for evidence Develop coping plans Change core beliefs	Worksheet 10.4 Chapters 4–7 Chapter 8 Chapter 9
Panic disorder	Catastrophic fears of physical or mental sensations	Identify specific fears Develop alternative Explanations for sensations Experiment to test fears	Chapter 5 Chapters 6, 7 Chapter 8
Phobias	Specific situational fears	Identify specific fear Look for evidence Develop a coping plan Exposure to fear with coping practice	Chapter 5 Chapters 6, 7 Chapter 8 Chapter 8
Obsessive-compulsive disorder	Intrusive thoughts are dangerous Thoughts make me responsible for whatever happens	Identify danger and responsibility beliefs Test beliefs about OCD thoughts Exposure to fears Response prevention	Chapter 5 Chapters 6, 7 Chapter 8 Chapter 8
Posttraumatic stress disorder	Thoughts about meaning of trauma Vulnerability thoughts Flashbacks Guilt-related thoughts Shame-related thoughts	Identify distressing meaning of trauma Look for survivorship meaning in trauma Develop coping plans (for flashbacks, too) Evaluate maladaptive core beliefs	Chapter 5 Chapters 6, 7 Chapter 8 Chapters 9, 12

RECOMMENDED READINGS

Barlow, D.H. (1988). *Anxiety and its disorders: The nature and treatment of anxiety and panic.* New York: Guilford Press.

Beck, A.T., Emery, G., & Greenberg, R.L. (1985). *Anxiety disorders and phobias: A cognitive perspective.* New York: Basic Books.

Hawton, K., Salkovskis, P.M., Kirk, J., & Clark, D.M. (Eds.). (1989). *Cognitive behaviour therapy for psychiatric problems: A practical guide.* New York: Oxford University Press.

Kennerley, H. (1995). *Managing anxiety: A training manual (2nd ed.).* New York: Oxford University Press.

Meichenbaum, D. (1994). *A clinical handbook/practical therapist manual for assessing and treating adults with post-traumatic stress disorder (PTSD).* Waterloo, Ontario: Institute Press.

Resick, P.A., & Schnicke, M.K. (1993). *Cognitive processing therapy for rape victims: A treatment manual.* Newbury Park, CA: Sage Publications.

Steketee, G.S. (1993). *Treatment of obsessive compulsive disorder.* New York: Guilford Press.

6

Using MIND OVER MOOD with Other Problems

Treatments for depression and anxiety disorders, detailed in Chapters 4 and 5 of this guide, are the most familiar applications of cognitive therapy. There are also cognitive models and treatment protocols for almost every type of client problem, as the recommended reading list at the end of this chapter shows. This chapter outlines general principles therapists can follow in adapting *Mind Over Mood* to accompany cognitive treatment of diverse client problems. We then illustrate the application of the principles in the treatment of substance abuse, eating disorders, relationship problems, and adjustment disorders.

GENERAL TREATMENT PRINCIPLES

To decide how to use the treatment manual in therapy for problems not specified in this clinician's guide, follow the steps in the Helpful Hints box on the following page. *Mind Over Mood* provides a framework to help clients learn skills that are essential to im-

107

proved psychological functioning. In evaluating clients, it is important to assess what strengths and attributes they possess as well as what skills need improvement. The treatment manual can help clients understand their problems better, identify feelings, identify thoughts, gather data that support and contradict beliefs, generate alternative views of situations, develop Action Plans and coping strategies, identify and test assumptions and core beliefs, and develop and test new assumptions and core beliefs. Most therapy protocols aim to help clients learn some or all of these skills to solve particular problems. Therefore, therapists are encouraged to assign treatment manual chapters that teach the skills of greatest help to a client. Use relevant chapters in the clinician's guide to troubleshoot problems that arise.

HELPFUL HINTS

Constructing Your Own Treatment Manual Protocols

When the clinician's guide does not provide a protocol for a particular client problem, ask yourself the following questions.

- **Is there a cognitive model for understanding and treating this problem?** If so, read relevant texts or articles to understand the treatment model and procedures (See the reference list at the end of this chapter). If not, construct a cognitive model for conceptualization and treatment using principles outlined in related texts (Beck et al., 1990; Freeman et al., 1989; Persons, 1989).

- **What skills does my client need to learn to successfully complete treatment?** Once you identify the skills, identify the chapters in *Mind Over Mood* that help teach the skills. Use the guidelines in Chapters 1 through 3 of the clinician's guide to assign the treatment manual chapters and troubleshoot difficulties encountered.

- **Are there personality factors that complicate treatment?** If so, follow the guidelines in Chapter 7 of this clinician's guide.

> • **Does the therapeutic response follow ex-
> pected patterns?** If not, formulate hypoth-
> eses for why client response is different from
> the expected response. Consider client be-
> liefs, skill deficits, emotional responses, inter-
> personal patterns, life circumstances, and
> developmental history. Also consider therapist
> beliefs, skill deficits, emotional responses;
> the therapy relationship (is it positive and
> collaborative?); the case conceptualization
> (is something missing or inaccurate?), and
> the treatment plan (are there additional ap-
> proaches that might help?).

SUBSTANCE ABUSE

Cognitive interventions designed to reduce substance abuse are
detailed in *Cognitive Therapy of Substance Abuse* (Beck, Wright,
Newman, & Liese, 1993). Cognitive therapy helps clients reduce
the frequency and severity of drinking or drug use by uncovering, examining, and altering the thoughts and beliefs that accompany urges to use. In addition, cognitive therapists teach coping
skills to addicted clients so that drug and alcohol use are replaced
with other strategies for managing moods, social situations, and
life problems.

The cognitive principles outlined in *Mind Over Mood* generally
can be taught in the order written when treating substance abus-
ing or addicted clients. Clients with substance abuse problems often avoid emotions. The basic information regarding identification
of moods in Chapter 3 of the treatment manual is important for
them to learn early in therapy. Once clients can identify moods,
they can learn to understand the causes of moods and new strategies for coping with their problems. Clients who do use alcohol
and drugs to numb mood are not very motivated to change their
behavior.

Early in therapy you should help your client identify beliefs
about the benefits of drugs and alcohol. For example, thoughts such
as "I need a drink to ease my pain," "I'll be more sociable if I have
some coke," or "I won't be able to cope if I don't use" are common

thoughts that accompany the urge to drink or use drugs. These thoughts can be identified, evaluated and eventually altered using the skills taught in Chapters 4 through 7 of *Mind Over Mood*. It is often helpful to set up collaborative behavioral experiments to evaluate these beliefs (Chapter 8) rather than simply arguing against drug or alcohol use.

———————————

Chris, a 21-year-old mechanic, entered therapy at the insistence of his parents who were concerned about his depression. At intake, Chris revealed that he was using cocaine nearly daily to cope with "bum moods." While Chris was willing to undergo treatment for depression, he did not want to discuss his cocaine habit because "it's not harmful; it's one of the few things that makes me feel better." When his therapist suggested that the cocaine might actually be contributing to his depression, Chris became defensive and said that it was not a problem for him and he didn't want to talk about it any more.

Following the guidelines for depression treatment outlined in Chapter 4 of this guide, Chris's therapist asked him to read the Prologue and Chapter 10 of *Mind Over Mood* to learn more about depression. Chris agreed to complete a Weekly Activity Schedule (Worksheet 10.4) to track his depressed mood. Since Chris felt cocaine was an important mood assist, his therapist suggested that he also mark his cocaine use on the Weekly Activity Schedule.

The data in the Weekly Activity Schedule Chris brought to the next appointment yielded several patterns. First, while Chris was depressed throughout the week, his mood ratings fluctuated considerably. Contrary to Chris's belief, cocaine use was not always followed by improved mood. Even when his mood was improved while on cocaine, Chris noticed that his depression always worsened several hours after snorting cocaine.

Although one week of data did not shift Chris's beliefs or willingness to stop using cocaine, the therapist persisted in using guided discovery to direct Chris's attention to some of the negative aspects of cocaine use. After four weeks of therapy, Chris was willing to begin doing experiments in which he reduced his cocaine use when depressed. He began identifying and testing beliefs associated with both depression and drug use following the guidelines in *Mind Over Mood*. Within another month, he was experimenting with prolonged abstinence from cocaine and was enjoying a noticeable decrease in depression. Eventually Chris stopped using cocaine entirely and also reduced his binge drinking to two or three beers on weekends, with a commitment to himself not to drink at all when he was depressed or upset.

Like Chris, many people who have a substance abuse problem also have mood or relationship problems. *Mind Over Mood* can be used as described in this guide to help people with substance abuse problems alleviate associated difficulties. Chapters 10 through 12 provide brief overviews to help clients understand depression, anxiety, anger, guilt, and shame, moods that commonly accompany substance abuse. The medication sections in Chapters 10 and 11 address addiction risk, a common concern of clients recovering from chemical dependency.

Some addicted clients have life problems (e.g., physical disabilities) or face social disadvantages (e.g., racial discrimination or high community unemployment rates) that seem hopeless to them. The problem-solving strategies described in Chapter 8 can help people begin to create Action Plans to cope with even the most difficult life circumstances. Extremely depressed clients with high levels of hopelessness need to be helped by their therapists to develop and carry out Action Plans.

As an example, an inner-city crack addict, Jim, had fewer internal and external resources than Chris, the employed mechanic who abused cocaine. A creative therapist was a powerful resource for Jim, helping him to come up with a small-steps plan for improvement. The first step was a medical detoxification program. The second was finding safe and drug-free housing. Over time, the therapist helped Jim enter a support group and find and maintain a job. The plans for changing Jim's life triggered both adaptive and maladaptive emotions and beliefs. The emotions and beliefs that interfered with progress were identified and tested using the strategies taught in Chapters 3 through 7 of *Mind Over Mood*.

Sometimes drug and alcohol abuse are associated with chronic low self-esteem or dysfunctional beliefs that maintain problems. Once clients have learned the skills taught in the first eight chapters of *Mind Over Mood*, these deeper core issues can be addressed following the strategies described in Chapter 9 of the treatment manual. Chapter 7 in this therapist's guide describes how to use Chapter 9 of the client manual to change core beliefs.

Relapse prevention is an important part of any substance abuse treatment program. The Action Plans described in Chapter 8 can be used to anticipate and plan for situations in which a client is at high risk to use alcohol or drugs. Many clients struggling with substance abuse or addiction identify with Vic, a recovering alcoholic described in *Mind Over Mood*. Chapters 6 and 7 of *Mind Over Mood* describe in detail how Vic used the manual's worksheets to prevent relapse drinking during a period of intense anger with his wife, Judy. In Chapter 8, clients can read how Vic set up an Action Plan to cope with his anger and improve his relationship with Judy while maintaining sobriety.

Mind Over Mood is compatible with 12-step programs including Alcoholics Anonymous (AA), Narcotics Anonymous, and Al-Anon as well as with inpatient and outpatient programs (e.g., Rational Recovery, S.M.A.R.T. Recovery) treating alcohol and drug dependency. Group treatment programs can use *Mind Over Mood* as a treatment guide for clients following the principles for group therapy outlined in Chapter 9 of the clinician's guide.

Twelve-step programs can select particular chapters from the treatment manual to help members successfully complete steps and avoid common pitfalls. For example, the fourth step in an AA program asks members to "make a searching and fearless moral inventory" and the fifth step directs members to admit wrongs to "God, to ourselves, and to another human being" (Alcoholics Anonymous, 1976, p. 59). Some AA members have an exaggerated response to these steps and blame themselves totally for every misfortune in life. Extreme self-blame can lead to overwhelming feelings of hopelessness and self-reproach, which in turn can increase a member's risk for renewed substance abuse.

Chapter 12 of the treatment manual helps 12-step program members understand and work with guilt and shame. Responsibility Pies (Worksheet 12.2) help AA members acknowledge responsibility without assigning excessive self-blame. This method is particularly helpful for women, who are prone to accepting excessive blame and responsibility for problems, ignoring other contributing factors.

REMINDER
BOX

Substance Abuse Treatment:
Mind Over Mood **Assignments**
- Prologue
- Chapters 1–3. Provide extra help if necessary for mood identification.
- Chapters 11, 12, or 13 if depression, anxiety, anger, guilt, or shame are predominant.
- Worksheet 10.4 (Weekly Activity Schedule.) Identify patterns of substance use, mood, and problem behaviors on Worksheet 10.5.
- Chapters 4–5 to help identify beliefs maintaining substance abuse and other problems.
- Chapters 6–7 to help evaluate beliefs.
- Chapter 8 for behavioral experiments to help evaluate beliefs maintaining substance abuse, for Action Plans to solve problems and develop new behavioral skills, and for relapse prevention.
- Chapter 9, if necessary, to evaluate core beliefs that maintain maladaptive beliefs and behaviors.

EATING DISORDERS

Fairburn (1985) and Garner and Bemis (1985) provide some of the clearest descriptions of cognitive therapy for eating disorders. Interested therapists can also read about this approach in the *Handbook of Psychotherapy for Anorexia Nervosa and Bulimia* (Garner & Garfinkel, 1985). All the skills taught in *Mind Over Mood* are useful for eating disorder clients. Clients with eating disorders should read the Prologue and then the portions of Chapters 10 through 12 that pertain to them. The remaining chapters can be read in the order written.

The one exception to this general guideline is that the Weekly Activity Schedule (Worksheet 10.4) is almost always helpful at the beginning of therapy for eating disorders. The Weekly Activity Schedule assesses the relationship between activity/behavior and mood. This worksheet can be modified for eating disorder clients to identify precipitants of increased levels of emotional distress, binging, purging, overeating, exercise, or other problems. Instruct clients to rate moods following the directions for this worksheet, and also to highlight with a star or other marker times when binging, purging, or other target behaviors occurred. Use Worksheet 10.5 to examine the connections among general behaviors and activities, eating disorder behaviors, and mood.

This assessment exercise is often followed by interventions that restructure activities to improve coping with precipitants of eating disorder behaviors. For example, one client with bulimia discovered that she binged and purged following weekly phone calls with her critical parents. She reduced her phone calls home and asked a trusted friend to sit with her during bi-monthly calls to offer her support and help counter negative thoughts that followed harsh parental criticism. As this client discovered, Action Plans (Chapter 8) that specify alternative coping strategies to binging, purging, and starvation are very helpful for eating disorder clients.

Like clients with substance abuse problems, clients with eating disorders often have difficulty identifying, differentiating, and rating emotions. Chapter 3 of the treatment manual can help clients attain these skills. Central to cognitive therapy of eating disorders, however, is restructuring of thought patterns that maintain the disorder. Chapters 4 through 7 teach clients to identify and test automatic thoughts, and Chapter 9 can be used to modify the deeper assumptions and core beliefs that are usually the center of the eating disorder storm.

Overeating and bulimia are usually easier to treat than anorexia nervosa. Clients with the first two disorders can usually perceive clear links between moods and impulsive eating behaviors. Once these clients learn to identify moods and delay eating behaviors to cope with these moods more directly, eating disorders diminish. For example, one client with bulimia learned to use her impulses to binge or purge as cues to look for the presence of an emotion. After learning to complete Thought Records, she used them to understand and work with her emotions prior to binging or purging. Most of the time, she felt better after completing a Thought Record. A reduction in emotional intensity made it easier for her to replace binging and purging with relaxation, assertion, or work on an Action Plan to solve an identified problem.

Clients with anorexa nervosa can also be treated with cognitive therapy, but they often demonstrate less emotional and cognitive awareness than bulimic clients, especially if the anorexia has progressed to the point of severe weight loss. Cognitive and emotional impairment are evident at very low body weight. Therapists focus on development of a positive and collaborative therapeutic relationship with low-weight anorexic clients rather than on teaching higher-level cognitive or emotional skills. If anorexic clients are strong enough to read and concentrate, they benefit from reading Chapters 1 through 3 and Chapters 10 through 12 of *Mind Over Mood* and completing the worksheets in these chapters.

Cognitive flexibility usually increases along with weight in clients with severe anorexia nervosa. Chapters 4 through 9 of the treatment manual are helpful to these clients when they gain enough weight to participate actively in psychotherapy. Common beliefs in anorexic clients include an assumption that self-worth is measured by body weight or shape, the conviction that complete self-control is desirable, and perfectionistic standards (Garner & Bemis, 1982, 1985). Therapists working with these sorts of beliefs are cautioned not to dispute them logically. Patient guided discovery with eating disorder clients is much more helpful than direct challenge of beliefs.

As an example, Cathy and her therapist identified two beliefs that were central to her anorexia nervosa: "I am as perfect as my weight" and "If I am not perfect, I am worthless." Since Cathy's idea of the perfect weight was so low it was medically dangerous, she needed to be hospitalized to regain weight she had lost. Then Cathy and her therapist used scales in Chapter 9 of the treatment manual and behavioral experiments in Chapter 8 to gradually shift Cathy's beliefs over an eight-month time period.

Cathy rated herself and others on her standards of perfection and discovered that she applied different weight rules to herself and to others. She also used rating scales to evaluate "perfection" and "worth" in a variety of areas of her life not directly tied to body weight. For example, she rated violin practice sessions on scales of perfection and worth. Cathy discovered that some practice sessions in which her playing was quite imperfect still had worth if she was able to learn something that improved her overall playing. Over time, Cathy began to see flaws in her underlying beliefs about perfection and worth. As she loosened perfectionism in other areas of her life, her concerns for maintaining a perfect weight also decreased.

Treatment of eating disorders can be straightforward or quite challenging. Treatment approaches require thorough knowledge of medical and psychosocial aspects of the disorder (for example, family patterns sometimes help maintain the problems) as well as the cognitive and behavioral components helped directly by the treatment manual.

REMINDER BOX

> **Eating Disorders:**
> *Mind Over Mood* **Assignments**
> * Prologue
> * Chapters 10–12: sections appropriate to understanding contributing moods.
> * Worksheet 10.4 (Weekly Activity Schedule). Identify patterns of general behaviors, moods, and eating behaviors.
> * Chapters 1–3. Provide extra help if necessary for mood identification.
> * Chapters 4–5 to help identify beliefs maintaining the eating disorder and other problems.
> * Chapters 6–7 to evaluate beliefs.
> * Chapter 8 for behavioral experiments to help evaluate beliefs maintaining eating disorder, for Action Plans to solve problems and develop new behavioral skills, and for relapse prevention.
> * Chapter 9 to evaluate core beliefs that maintain maladaptive behaviors.

RELATIONSHIP PROBLEMS

Cognitive therapy helps couples identify the beliefs and expectations that underlie anger and disappointment in their relationships (Baucom & Epstein, 1990; Dattilio & Padesky, 1990). *Love Is Never Enough* (Beck, 1988), written for couples, describes how unspoken expectations can turn hopeful love into bitter anger. The case examples in this book show readers how to evaluate and modify thoughts that maintain relationship discontent. Together, *Mind Over Mood* and *Love Is Never Enough* provide a complete therapy supplement for couples in cognitive therapy. Whereas the latter book describes the evolution of relationship conflict and recommended solutions, the treatment manual provides couples with detailed explanations and worksheets to help each person identify feelings, thoughts, and trouble spots in the relationship.

Cognitive therapy with couples has nine stages: (1) conceptualization of the couple's problems based on history, (2) crisis management for destructive anger, (3) increasing positive interactive behaviors, (4) helping the couple learn to identify, test, and respond to problem-related automatic thoughts, (5) communications skills training, (6) exploration of issues underlying anger, (7) teaching problem resolution strategies, (8) identifying and changing maladaptive core beliefs, and (9) relapse prevention (Dattilio & Padesky, 1990, pp. 76–77). The treatment manual can help couples successfully complete each of these stages. Couples who struggle with identification of feelings can read Chapter 3. Chapter 12 provides couples with a concise overview of anger, guilt, and shame, three of the most common feelings reported during relationship difficulties. Chapters 4–7 help couples build skills for identifying and testing the silent thoughts that add to relationship distress by interfering with communication, fueling anger, and blocking positive interactions. Chapter 8 teaches strategies for solving problems and experimenting with new relationship behaviors.

A couple can learn many of the basic skills taught in the treatment manual outside the therapy hour, freeing the therapist to spend more session time helping the couple understand and change relationship difficulties. Many relationship difficulties stem from dysfunctional core beliefs (e.g., "Men can't understand women," "The mother is solely responsible for child care," "True love means accepting me as I am," "Anger is always damaging"). Chapter 9 of the treatment manual supports the work being done in therapy sessions by helping couples identify and examine the core beliefs.

It is ideal for both partners to work on core beliefs. If only one partner is doing this more intensive therapy work, the couple may conclude that this partner is more responsible for the relationship problems. All people have maladaptive core beliefs that are activated at times in their closest relationships. When awareness of maladaptive core beliefs is increased and the beliefs are replaced with balanced core beliefs, relationships thrive. If a couple does not show punitive or destructive patterns, each partner can support core belief change in the other by pointing out information to be recorded on the Core Belief Records (Worksheets 9.5 and 9.6).

As an example, Jane and Wanda sought therapy when they began to experience increased conflict in their five-year relationship. Frequent fights were fueled by Jane's underlying assumption "If she loves me, she'll know [and do] what I want" and Wanda's core belief "People in love don't criticize or fight." A pattern of conflict developed: (1) Jane felt hurt when Wanda did not anticipate her unspoken needs. (2) Jane expressed this hurt by making small critical comments to Wanda. (3) Wanda interpreted Jane's criticism as a sign that Jane didn't love her anymore. (4) Wanda withdrew from Jane, feeling certain that the relationship was ending. (5) Jane became angrier, as Wanda's attention to her decreased, until she finally exploded in anger. (6) Wanda cried in response to Jane's anger, saying she still loved Jane and didn't want to break up. (7) Jane was puzzled, saying she loved Wanda and only wanted Wanda to remain connected and involved. (8) Wanda felt relieved that Jane did love her and paid Jane increased positive attention during the ensuing days. (9) The relationship conflict was resolved until the next time these issues surfaced.

This couple improved when the therapist charted this pattern on a piece of paper and asked each woman to examine the core belief that contributed to her portion of the conflict. Jane recognized logically that Wanda might not always know what Jane wanted unless Jane directly communicated her wishes. However, she discovered that this core belief was activated anyway when she was emotionally tired and most prone to irritability.

On core belief worksheets, Jane noted data that contradicted her belief. For example, Jane realized that as much as she loved Wanda, she often did not have a clue to what would please Wanda in a given moment. Jane interviewed friends and discovered that they also frequently misunderstood their partner's needs when the needs were not explicitly expressed. In therapy sessions, Wanda helped Jane understand that her love was deep but not omniscient.

In turn, Wanda examined her own core belief "People in love don't criticize or fight." She interviewed friends in good relationships and discovered that they all fought and criticized sometimes. She worked on developing an alternative core belief, "People who are in love use fights and criticism to improve their relationship." To test this new perspective, Wanda tried to fight constructively in conflicts with Jane instead of withdrawing. During conflicts in session, the therapist coached Wanda to help her remain active, listening to Jane's concerns and expressing her own. In time, Wanda and Jane each developed more adaptive core beliefs that supported interactive conflict resolution. New beliefs and skills gained in therapy and supported by the treatment manual helped them restore a mutually loving relationship.

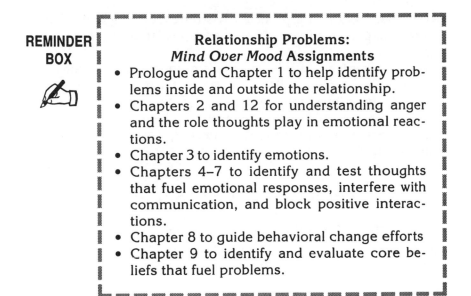

REMINDER
BOX

Relationship Problems:
***Mind Over Mood* Assignments**
- Prologue and Chapter 1 to help identify problems inside and outside the relationship.
- Chapters 2 and 12 for understanding anger and the role thoughts play in emotional reactions.
- Chapter 3 to identify emotions.
- Chapters 4–7 to identify and test thoughts that fuel emotional responses, interfere with communication, and block positive interactions.
- Chapter 8 to guide behavioral change efforts
- Chapter 9 to identify and evaluate core beliefs that fuel problems.

ADJUSTMENT DISORDERS

Often people seek therapy for help with distress that follows recent life stresses or changes. Cognitive therapy is helpful for adjustment disorders. Therapists treating clients with adjustment difficulties are encouraged to structure *Mind Over Mood* use to meet clients' immediate individual needs. Follow the guidelines for constructing individualized treatment protocols in the Helpful Hints box on pages 108–109. Construct a model with the client for understanding his or her problem(s) and how life events and their meanings for the client triggered problems (Persons, 1989).

Next, consider what skills are necessary to help the client navigate this challenging time in his or her life. Some clients may not know how to identify their emotions and may initially benefit most from Chapter 3 (Identifying and Rating Moods). Other people are fully aware of what they are feeling and capable of articulating their feelings. For these clients, Chapter 3 can be eliminated or skimmed.

Many clients wonder why a certain change or event has been so distressing when they have managed other problems in their life with ease. These clients can use Chapter 5 to help identify their thoughts about the event. Understanding an event's meaning often provides useful clues regarding the importance of the event to the client and reasons for particularly strong reactions to it. Chapter 8 will help clients if an Action Plan is required to solve problems.

Refer to Chapter 7 of this clinician's guide for suggestions on how to use Chapters 8 and 9 in the treatment manual to work with lifelong dysfunctional core beliefs and behavior patterns if they play an important role in the presenting problem. Chapter 7 also includes hints for resolving problems that might arise in the therapy relationship.

RECOMMENDED READINGS

In lieu of a Troubleshooting Guide for this chapter, we offer a bibliography of texts and reference materials to help therapists conceptualize and construct protocols for the diverse client problems that can be helped with *Mind Over Mood*.

Baucom, D., & Epstein, N. (1990). *Cognitive-behavioral marital therapy.* New York: Brunner/Mazel.

Beck, A.T. (1988). *Love is never enough.* New York: Harper & Row.

Beck, A.T., Wright, F.D., Newman, C.F., & Liese, B.S. (1993). *Cognitive therapy of substance abuse.* New York: Guilford Press.

Dattilio, F.M., & Padesky, C. A. (1990). *Cognitive therapy with couples.* Sarasota, FL: Professional Resource Exchange.

Epstein, N., Schlesinger, S., & Dryden W. (1988). *Cognitive-behavioral therapy with families.* New York: Brunner/Mazel.

Freeman, A., & Dattilio, F.M. (Eds.). (1992). *Comprehensive casebook of cognitive therapy.* New York: Plenum Press.

Freeman, A., Simon, K.M., Beutler, L. E., & Arkowitz, H. (Eds.). (1989). *Comprehensive handbook of cognitive therapy.* New York: Plenum Press.

Garner, D.M., & Garfinkel, P.E. (Eds.). (1985). *Handbook of psychotherapy for anorexia nervosa and bulimia.* New York: Guilford Press.

Golden, W.L., Gersh, W.D., & Robbins, D.M. (1992). *Psychological treatment of cancer patients: A cognitive-behavioral approach.* Boston: Allyn and Bacon.

Kingdon, D.G., & Turkington, D. (1994). *Cognitive-behavioral therapy of schizophrenia.* New York: Guilford Press.

Scott, J., Williams, J.M.G., & Beck, A.T. (Eds.). (1989). *Cognitive therapy in clinical practice: An illustrative casebook.* New York: Routledge.

7

Using MIND OVER MOOD with Personality Disorders

Many clients who seek therapy for depression, anxiety and the other presenting problems described in Chapters 4 through 6 of this guide also meet diagnostic criteria for personality disorders (Axis II of DSM-IV). Clients with Axis II disorders and even some with long-term Axis I disorders (e.g., long-term dysthymia) can be differentiated from clients with short-term difficulties by the presence of strongly held negative core beliefs, or schemas. While all of us have schemas, including maladaptive schemas, the maladaptive schemas of clients with lifelong problems are believed to maintain their difficulties because they are not balanced by the presence of adaptive schemas (Padesky, 1994a).

Cognitive theory hypothesizes that schemas are formed in response to real developmental circumstances (e.g., growing up with manipulative, damaging others) and/or biological influences rather than from gross distortions of experience. Most of us develop both

121

positive and negative schemas regarding our self (e.g., "I'm competent," "I'm incompetent"), others (e.g., "People can be trusted," "People can't be trusted"), and the world (e.g., "The world is overwhelming," "The world is manageable"). These schemas are differentially activated depending on mood (e.g., when depressed our self-critical, hopeless schemas emerge; when happy, our more positive self, other, and world schemas emerge), circumstance (e.g., in a dangerous neighborhood, schemas of vulnerability emerge; at home, schemas of safety emerge), recent life events (e.g., following trauma, schemas of vulnerability and mistrust emerge), and even biology (e.g., physiological activation, fatigue, and illness can influence schema activation).

According to cognitive theory, clients with Axis II disorders hold negative schemas in certain domains without a well-developed companion positive schema (Padesky, 1988, 1994a). These clients maintain certain schematic views regardless of mood, circumstance, life events, or biological state. For example, a client with dependent personality disorder sees himself as weak even following a personal mastery experience. A client with avoidant personality disorder views herself as inadequate even when she is valued as a mother by her children, loved by her husband, and regularly promoted in her job.

Although negative schemas may not be the cause of personality disorders, they serve a powerful maintenance function (Padesky, 1994a). Negative schemas emerge in the therapy relationship and can lead to noncompliance factors (e.g., "I'm a failure. What's the use in trying anything new?") or relationship difficulties (e.g., "I can't trust anyone. You'll hurt me, too."). Negative schemas interfere with client ability to recognize progress (e.g., "Oh sure, I was promoted in my job, but that's just because my boss doesn't see the real me"), accept positive feedback (e.g., "You have to say that because you're my therapist"), or learn from setbacks (e.g., "Of course it didn't work out. I'm no good. There's no reason to problem solve and try again").

According to schema theory, we can perceive only what our schemas prepare us to see. Life experiences that contradict our activated schema are discounted, distorted, not noticed, or viewed as an exception to broader "reality" (Padesky, 1993b). Therefore, if we have paired schemas ("I am lovable," "I am not lovable"), we are capable of perceiving and remembering both positive and negative reactions from other people. However, if we hold only the negative schema for certain areas of our life, we are able to perceive and remember only experiences in that domain insofar as we fit them to our schema. For example, a woman who believes "I'm unlovable" without the companion schema "I'm lovable" perceives every human interaction as proof of her unlovability. Negative responses from others fit her schema perfectly. Positive reactions from others are not noticed or distorted ("She is so kind to act nice toward me, even though I probably disgust her"), discounted ("He probably says this to everyone"), or seen as an exception ("Oh, sure, she likes me now. But when she gets to know the real me she'll see how unlovable I am").

Beck and his colleagues (1990) specify schemas that seem to maintain each of the personality disorders and articulate treatment plans for each disorder. As described in their book, cognitive therapy of personality disorders involves using the therapy relationship as a schema laboratory in which the client can safely evaluate maladaptive core beliefs. The developmental origins of schemas are explored so that the client can understand the circumstances under which the schemas are adaptive and learn to recognize when life circumstances allow alternative schemas to be safely held. The therapy hinges on weakening client conviction that negative schemas are always true and constructing alternative schemas so that the client can perceive and accept positive as well as negative data (Padesky, 1994a). Behavioral experiments designed to practice more adaptive behavior patterns and to test the utility of alternative schemas also are central to the therapy.

Can a treatment manual be helpful for these clients? If it can, does it need to be introduced or used any differently? How does *Mind Over Mood* fit with the cognitive therapy treatment of personality disorders described by Beck and colleagues (1990)? This chapter suggests strategies for using *Mind Over Mood* to (1) assist treatment of Axis I clinical disorders or psychosocial problems in clients with personality disorders and (2) change core schemas and problematic behavior patterns when the focus of treatment is the personality disorder itself.

CAN A TREATMENT MANUAL BE HELPFUL FOR CLIENTS WITH PERSONALITY DISORDERS?

Early versions of *Mind Over Mood* were used in inpatient group therapy with a population that included a high percentage of patients with severe depression and concurrent Axis II diagnoses, especially borderline personality disorder. These patients were enthusiastic about using a treatment manual in their program. Many experienced extreme fluctuations in mood and had little experience identifying and evaluating their reactions. The manual helped them organize and understand their experiences better. Written summaries in the manual helped these patients learn the ideas presented in group therapy more quickly.

Clients with personality disorders in outpatient psychotherapy who use the current version of *Mind Over Mood* similarly report on feedback forms that the treatment manual is very helpful. Since clients with Axis II disorders have long-term patterns that are difficult to change, written records help organize and integrate new learning. For example, one client kept a notebook for three years and referred to it whenever he became depressed. He reported that review of Thought Records and core belief worksheets he had written during previous depressions helped prevent current depressed moods from worsening.

Clients who have difficulty in direct interpersonal relationships find that the treatment manual provides a private forum for experimentation with new ideas. For example, avoidant clients sometimes find it helpful to practice new ideas on paper until they have the courage to describe them aloud to a therapist. Further, clients who benefit from repetition can practice exercises at their own speed and review completed worksheets to reinforce learning. One woman with borderline personality disorder found that she could delay impulsive behavior by identifying and rating her feelings as taught in Chapter 3 of the treatment manual. She read and reread Chapter 3 whenever she experienced overwhelming emotion.

INTRODUCING *MIND OVER MOOD* TO CLIENTS WITH PERSONALITY DISORDERS

The same guidelines offered in Chapter 1 of this guide regarding introduction of a treatment manual into therapy pertain to clients with personality disorders. It is important to provide a rationale for its use, link the treatment manual to achievement of client goals, allow time to discuss how the manual will be used in therapy, give clear instructions on how to use it, and ask the client to bring *Mind Over Mood* to therapy sessions. Therapist interest in maximizing client learning should be emphasized.

Implementation of the standard principles goes smoothly with most clients with personality disorders. Occasionally, however, the introduction of a treatment manual, like other therapy procedures, will trigger idiosyncratic client responses that need to be addressed. Several possible client reactions are described along with recommendations for dealing with them in a manner that enhances rather than disrupts the therapy relationship. For a more thorough discussion of client reactions to therapy procedures and therapeutic responses based on a cognitive conceptualization of personality disorders, read *Cognitive Therapy of Personality Disorders* (Beck et al., 1990); the book presents a cognitive conceptualization and treatment plan for each personality disorder.

Avoidant Responses

Some clients are afraid to reveal their innermost thoughts and feelings in therapy. Their fears are often the result of previous traumatic interpersonal experiences. Avoidant clients often hold beliefs such as "People will reject me if I let them know who I am," "I'm a failure," "I'm unimportant," "It's dangerous to say too much," "My thoughts are crazy." It is not surprising that clients who hold these beliefs are hesitant to show a therapist written exercises detailing thoughts and emotional reactions to events in their lives. These clients may compliantly agree to use *Mind Over Mood* and then "forget" to bring it to session or refuse to show written exercises to the therapist. The following vignette illustrates one way to handle this client response.

T: Did you bring *Mind Over Mood* for discussion today?

C: No, I forgot it.

T: You forgot it last week, too. I wonder if there is some reason you are not bringing it here.

C: No, I just forgot.

T: It's certainly possible to forget. Yet I've learned that sometimes clients are hesitant to bring their books in. Can you imagine why?

C: No.

T: Well, some don't like to use the book. Others use the book but don't feel comfortable showing me what they've written. Others have very personal reasons for not bringing the book. What has been your experience so far?

C: What do you mean?

T: Well, first of all, do you like the book?

C: Yes. It's helpful.

T: Have you done any of the written exercises?

C: Yes, some of them.

T: How would you feel if you showed them to me?

C: I guess a little uncomfortable.

T: What would be uncomfortable?

C: I don't know. Maybe your reactions.

T: What kind of reactions do you imagine I might have?

C: You might be disappointed in me.

T: Hmm. What would I be disappointed about?

C: If I didn't do it right. Or if my thoughts are pretty screwy.

T: And if I were disappointed that you didn't do it right or I thought you had screwy thoughts, then what would happen?

C: You'd be disgusted with me.

T: And then . . . ?

C: (*Red-faced, looking into lap*) You'd get angry with me and not be my therapist any more.

T: Do you have an image of that in your mind right now?

(*Client nods.*)

T: How are you feeling right now?

C: Ashamed.

T: Does this feeling and image remind you of anything?

C: (*Downcast and teary-eyed*) How I felt when my father stood me up against the wall and yelled at me when I made a mistake.

T: (*Slowly and quietly*) Hearing how you'd expect me to react really helps me understand why you would be hesitant to bring in your book and show me your exercises. Let's spend some time today talking about this mental picture of me, the memory of your father, and how we can handle things so it's not so risky for you to bring your book to session.

C: OK.

This vignette illustrates steps that can be taken to identify the feelings and beliefs that can interfere with use of *Mind Over Mood* in therapy. First the therapist asks the client directly and noncritically if anything is interfering with bringing the manual to session. When the client says no, the therapist provides some examples of reasons that might contribute to a hesitancy to bring the book to the session. A range of reasons shows the client he or she is not alone and that there are good reasons for noncompliance. Guiding questions are asked to help the client identify feelings and the thoughts (including images and memories) accompanying these feelings. Finally, the therapist empathizes with the client's reasons to show understanding and foster a collaborative review of these beliefs and reactions.

In the example the therapist skillfully elicits beliefs and emotional reactions that interfere with using the treatment manual as fully as possible in therapy. At times, the therapist can inadvertently be partially responsible for the client's reactions. For example, if the therapist asks to see the treatment manual abruptly, the client's fears of punishment may be exacerbated. If the therapist contributes to client fears, the therapist can help restore collaboration by acknowledging his or her role in eliciting a negative client response.

Once the difficulties are understood by both therapist and client, strategies for resolving them can be discussed. For example, some avoidant clients appreciate the opportunity to read small portions of worksheets to the therapist and to discuss the therapist's reactions before revealing more information. Other clients are willing to reveal thoughts and feelings only after the therapist has shown how a range of reactions are seen as normal.

Generally, a small-steps approach is taken with avoidant clients to allow gradual revelation of thoughts and feelings and give ample attention to discussing therapist and client reactions to these internal events. Risks taken by clients in the therapy relationship are viewed as behavioral experiments and can be set up as described in Chapter 8 of *Mind Over Mood* . It is important to ask for a client's prediction of what consequence will follow these interpersonal risks, discuss strategies for overcoming any hazards that might occur, and discuss the actual outcome of self-revelation. Avoidant clients commonly predict rejection, criticism, or intense negative emotions and in reality experience a sense of relief or even acceptance once they have described their inner experience. A therapist can underscore that, although negative outcomes may have been the norm in a client's past, therapy will offer a chance to learn what circumstances and relationships are safe for self-expression.

HELPFUL HINTS

Therapeutic Responses to Negative Client Reactions to *Mind Over Mood*

- Expect core beliefs to emerge in response to the treatment manual.
- Ask for feedback directly.
- Explore negative reactions and adopt a curious, open attitude.
- Help the client identify thoughts and feelings.
- Ask for memories and images to look for similarities with past experiences.
- Empathize with and summarize your understanding of the client's negative reactions.
- Acknowledge any portion of the disruption in collaboration for which you are responsible.
- Collaboratively explore solutions to identified problems.
- Set up and conduct behavioral experiments.
- Debrief the outcome of behavioral experiments; comparing it with predictions; problem solve further if necessary.

Suspicious Responses

Some clients respond to *Mind Over Mood* or other therapy interventions with suspicion. These clients hold beliefs such as "Information I give you will be used to hurt me," "No one can be trusted," "I must be on guard at all times, " "People have hidden motives." Some suspicious clients may ask the therapist not to keep any written records of sessions. The same strategies outlined in the section on avoidant responses and the Helpful Hints box above can be used with these clients, who may be even more reluctant than avoidant clients to reveal beliefs and emotional reactions.

First, the therapist can normalize mistrust and suspiciousness by validating a client's concerns: "I can understand your hesitation. After all, I'm a stranger to you. Just because I have a diploma on my wall doesn't mean you can trust me." Trust is not achieved through assurances but rather through direct and open communication. For example, it is helpful to clarify the purposes for which the treatment manual and other therapy procedures will be used.

This manual is designed to help you practice the skills you learn in therapy. If you want to keep your worksheets private, that is your choice. I will encourage you, however, to show them to me because it will help us work together if we both know what problems and successes you are having. You can make decisions about showing me your worksheets as you get to know me better.

I will keep written records of our sessions because it is my professional obligation to do so. The written records ensure that I am following a treatment plan with you, help me remember important information related to solving your problems, and provide a record if you ever want or need to have a summary of what we did together. You are welcome to look at your written file with me any time you like.

Thus, the therapist expresses genuine empathy by acknowledging that the client has little information by which to judge the therapist's trustworthiness. By offering information in a nondefensive manner, the therapist conveys respect for the client's concerns. A therapist who verbally reassures ("You can trust me") or becomes argumentative about procedures ("If you want to work with me, you have to show me your worksheets") will exacerbate suspiciousness.

As with avoidance, therapist and client need to develop strategies for solving the problems posed by client beliefs. Behavioral experiments can be designed to explore trust in the relationship. Rather than viewing trust as an all-or-nothing phenomenon, therapists can ask clients to consider what type and degree of information they think they can safely share with the therapist. Some clients choose to state beliefs and emotional reactions for some areas of their life but not others. For example, one client would talk about his feelings of betrayal in relationships but refused to describe the thoughts and images related to his anger.

It is important to allow these boundaries to exist if the client so chooses. In the case of the man who would not reveal his angry thoughts, his therapist allowed these thoughts to remain private. However, the therapist discussed philosophical beliefs about anger and violence with the client. While respecting the client's privacy, the therapist was able to defuse violent impulses by reaching agreement with the client about the undesirable risks of violence (e.g., he could be imprisoned) and by teaching strategies for assertively managing situations that triggered anger.

Angry Responses

Some clients respond to *Mind Over Mood* with anger. When this happens, it is important to uncover the beliefs or other emotions that fuel the anger. Some clients respond with anger when mistrust is triggered, similar to the suspicious clients. Other clients become angry following the activation of hurt or fear. For example, a client might think, "She's giving me a book to use because she doesn't want to have to talk to me" or "This book is a way of telling me it's time to terminate therapy." Other reasons for anger are the perception of a violation of rights or a sense of belittlement: "He's telling me my problems aren't important," "I'm just like someone in a book to her; she doesn't see me as special," or "I'm just going to receive a standard book; no attention will be paid to me as an individual."

Following the principles in the Helpful Hint box on page 128 of this guide, therapists can adopt a curious, nondefensive posture and show interest in understanding the beliefs and emotions connected to anger. Whereas gentle encouragement characterizes the therapeutic response to avoidance and direct information is offered to the suspicious client, the angry client often requires a calm, direct, open curiosity from the therapist, as illustrated in the following session excerpt.

C: I can't believe you're asking me to read a book!

T: What do you mean?

C: (*Mocking*) "What do you mean?" Don't be a jerk.

T: You seem really ticked off at me. I'm serious when I say I'm not sure why.

C: How would you feel if your therapist gave you a book?

T: I think it would depend on why I thought she was giving me the book.

C: Exactly!

T: I guess I'm a bit slow today. I'm not sure why you think I asked you to read this book.

C: It's clear. You're fed up with me and are ready to pack me off to the self-help section of the bookstore.

T: So you think I'm giving you this book to get you to stop coming to therapy?

C: (*Raising voice*) Oh, don't act so innocent! I knew you'd get sick of me. You're not the first therapist to be fed up with me. I just thought you'd have a little class and tell me directly. Well, I quit! (*Stands up to leave office.*)

T: Wait a minute! Slow down. You're reading me wrong. Please sit down for a few more minutes to sort this out.

(*Client sits reluctantly.*)

T: I'm not giving you this book to get rid of you or abandon you to self-help. In my experience, this book is very helpful to people while they are in therapy. I wanted you to try it in addition to seeing me.

C: Why? Don't you think you can help me?

T: I think I can help you better if we have a written summary of our work together. This manual helps us create a summary.

C: I've read lots of books. They never help.

T: This book is a little different. You don't just read it. You use it as a guide for learning and practicing skills that might help you feel more in control of your moods.

C: "Might?" You mean it might not help at all?

T: Of course that's a possibility. I do think it will help you, but it may not. We won't know unless you give it a try. And I'll be here to help you figure out any parts that don't make sense to you. We'll use the book together.

C: You really think it might help?

In this example, the therapist needs to quickly identify the client's beliefs before anger terminates the therapy relationship. Once the client's beliefs are uncovered, the therapist directly addresses them. Note that the therapist does not guarantee that the manual will be helpful; using the manual is again presented as a behavioral experiment.

It is important to help clients with frequent anger identify the common triggers of this response. For example, one client learned that she became angry when she felt threatened. She used the anger to defend herself against an anticipated attack. Once she realized the pattern, she was able to use her anger as a cue to look for automatic thoughts and images regarding risk for attack. Learning the skills in chapters 6 and 7 of *Mind Over Mood* helped her evaluate these situations more quickly, and she began to experience less anger in the many situations in which she decided threat was not imminent.

TREATING AXIS I PROBLEMS IN CLIENTS WITH CONCURRENT AXIS II DIAGNOSES

Despite researchers' expectations, several studies have shown that clients with concurrent Axis II diagnoses do as well in cognitive therapy for depression and anxiety as clients without concurrent Axis II diagnoses (Arntz & Dreessen, 1990; Dreessen, Arntz, Luttels, & Sallaerts, 1994; Dreessen, Hoekstra & Arntz, 1995; Emanuels-Zuurveen & Emmelkamp, 1995; Van Velzen & Emmelkamp, 1995). Therefore, it is reasonable to follow the treatment protocols outlined in Chapters 4 and 5 even if a client meets criteria for personality disorders as well.

Some clients with personality disorders require no modifications in how the treatment manual is used for treating Axis I problems. Other clients benefit most if manual use is modified for (1) the therapy relationship, (2) the therapy pace, (3) the client's repetition needs and/or (4) order of topic presentation. Clinical examples illustrating the necessity and use of these modifications follow.

Therapy Relationship

Schemas central to Axis II diagnoses are often expressed most clearly in the therapy relationship. Clients with avoidant personality disorder believe that the therapist sees them as inferior and inadequate; clients with obsessive–compulsive personality disorder try to do every task perfectly and are loathe to depend on the therapist for help; clients with narcissistic personality disorder constantly scan for indications that the therapist thinks they are special and demand attention when they feel vulnerable.

Each of these client types responds quite differently to use of a treatment manual. And in different ways, the therapy relationship can be used to foster manual use for each client. For example, the avoidant client requires extra reassurance, therapist support, and behavioral experiments in self-revelation, as illustrated in the therapist–client dialogue on pages 125–126.

Clients with obsessive–compulsive personality disorder (OCPD) are usually eager to use the manual, although they may criticize limitations or errors found in it. With these clients, the manual can provide a forum for testing beliefs such as "Unless I do things perfectly, they have no value" and "I am fully responsible for everything." The therapist can challenge the client to use the manual to test some of these beliefs. For example, the therapist can ask a client with OCPD to complete some of the worksheets partially or imperfectly and see if they still have learning value. Also, the therapist can use the manual to illustrate a midpoint on the continuum between complete self-reliance to complete dependence on others. The therapy relationship and the treatment manual are geared to help the client while he or she also helps him or herself. This balance of help and independence appeals to most clients with OCPD and can help them begin to relinquish a need to be in complete control of the therapy.

Clients with narcissistic personality disorders may balk at the use of a standardized treatment manual. A core schematic belief for these clients is "I am worthless if I am not special." Therapist introduction of a treatment manual can therefore trigger the worthlessness schema and coping behavior that protect the client from the depressed feelings this schema engenders. Coping behaviors may include (a) making demeaning statements about the therapist ("You must be new at this if you have to use a book"), (b) assertions of specialness ("I'll have you know that I always get personal service, and if you expect me to follow a program like a trained seal, I'll take my business elsewhere"), and (c) appealing to the therapist's own narcissism ("I'm sure I could learn this better and faster from you than from a book. Why don't we just talk this through like two intelligent people?").

Responses such as these provide opportunities to identify the worthlessness schema and use the therapy relationship to begin treatment of the narcissistic personality itself. The therapist does this by deflecting attack and empathically searching for the worthless core. Possible therapist responses to narcissistic coping behaviors are (a) "I wonder if the idea of using a book like this triggers some feelings in you?" or "You must feel somewhat discouraged that I think a book like this would help you, given the depth of your feelings," (b) "Introducing this book seems to make you feel as if I don't see you as very special. Does that make you feel anything besides anger?" and (c) "What would it be like for you to read and learn from a book, without the attention you receive from me when we meet face to face?" Note that each of these therapist responses asks the client to focus on feelings, especially the types of feelings the client with narcissistic personality disorder wishes to avoid, such as depression and loneliness.

These examples illustrate how use of the manual triggers relationship issues in therapy. Many of the personality disorders produce a signature response to the manual, which is predicted by the schema beliefs central to the disorder. For example, relative to other clients, those with dependent personality disorder request much more help from the therapist to complete *Mind Over Mood* exercises and seek reassurance that the manual is not a replacement for the therapist's assistance. These responses to manual use highlight relationship issues early in therapy, so the therapist can begin to therapeutically respond to them at an early date. For more specific guidelines for how to use the therapy relationship to help clients with personality disorders, see Beck and colleagues (1990).

Therapy Pace

Some clients with Axis II disorders require individualized adjustments in the pace at which the treatment manual is used. Clients with avoidant personality disorder (AvPD) prefer not to think about painful thoughts and emotions, so the manual may become a symbol of what is "unpleasant" about therapy to them. These clients are more likely to use the manual if given timed assignments in the manual followed by pleasant activities. For example, the therapist may recommend 10 or 15 minutes of manual use prior to watching a favorite TV show. As AvPD clients become more familiar with experiencing emotions and the skills for managing them, they will be more willing to use the manual for longer periods of time.

In contrast, some clients with borderline personality disorder (BPD) benefit most if they use the manual several times a day. These clients experience frequent mood swings and can use Chapter 3 of *Mind Over Mood* to identify and rate their moods and later chapters of the book to help modulate them. Some clients with BPD need to follow a slow pace through the manual, spending several weeks on chapters that teach skills for which they have particular need. The therapist can help these clients by encouraging them to take as much time as necessary to master component skills.

Repetition Needs of the Client

Many clients read *Mind Over Mood* and add to their skill repertoire chapter by chapter with little need to refer to earlier worksheets or summaries. Others require frequent repetition of skills to master them. All clients with personality disorders (as well as those with chronic problems) need repetition once they begin the core belief work described in Chapter 9 of *Mind Over Mood* and illustrated later in this chapter of the clinician's guide. Repetition is necessary to promote development of new schemas because schemas generally change quite slowly.

In addition, since schemas are core to many of the automatic thoughts and underlying assumptions of clients with Axis II diagnoses, earlier chapters of *Mind Over Mood* may also require more repetition. For example, a client with major depression and no personality disorder may recover completely after learning the skills in the manual and completing 15 or 20 thought records and five or six behavioral experiments. For this client, the skills practice restores the more balanced thinking style characteristic of his or her nondepressed state.

In comparison, a client with major depression and BPD may learn the skills in the manual in a comparable period of time and experience a lifting of the major depression. Yet this client may not experience a stable restoration of balanced thinking because, in many domains of his or her life, negative schemas are characteristic of the nondepressed as well as depressed state. This client would therefore benefit from ongoing repetition of the worksheets in the manual along with ongoing schema change efforts as outlined later in this chapter of the clinician's guide.

Order of Topic Presentation

If clients hold schemas that strongly interfere with learning skills in the early chapters of *Mind Over Mood*, it may be advisable to introduce principles from Chapter 9 early in therapy. For example, Joan had great difficulty testing her automatic thoughts because each one seemed 100% true to her and no amount of data convinced her that her perceptions of situations were perceptions rather than truth. Joan's therapist suggested that Joan temporarily stop using Thought Records and instead use a scale (as described in Chapter 9 of *Mind Over Mood*) to rate her conclusions in problem situations. The following dialogue shows how this change in the order of skill mastery was helpful to Joan.

T: So when Patty got angry with you, you "knew" she hated you.

J: That's right. And I don't need to deal with that. So I broke up with her. And that's why I didn't have anything to write in the "Evidence That Does Not Support the Hot Thought" column. It was true.

T: Let's take a somewhat different approach to see if we can understand this better. Remember how you learned to rate feelings from 0 to 100%?

J: Yeah, sure.

T: Let's use a 0 to 100% scale to rate your conclusion "Patty hates me."

J: OK. 100% true.

T: (*Drawing a scale from 0 to 100%*) Here's the line to measure how much someone hates you. Now, you put an "X" where you think Patty's feelings lie.

(*Joan draws an "X" at 100%.*)

T: Let's clarify. Does 100% mean the most anyone can hate you?

J: Yes.

T: So you can't imagine anyone hating you as much as you're sure Patty does.

J: No. That's why I was so upset! After all we've been through together, it made me so mad she turned on me like that.

T: What if someone hated you so much they physically assaulted you or killed you? Where would that go on this continuum?

J: I guess that would be 100%.

T: And Patty reacted to you that violently?

J: No. Of course not.

T: I want to make sure this scale includes all of your possible experience. So let's put violence on the scale and rate it. Have you ever been victim of this kind of hate?

J: Yes. Once I was beaten up outside a gay bar.

T: I'm so sorry. (*Pauses.*) Where would you put that kind of experience on this hate scale?

J: That would be 100%.

T: Any other hate experiences you've had that could go on this scale?

J: My uncle molested me. That wasn't actually as hateful as the bar thing. But it sure wasn't loving.

T: Where would you put that on this scale?

J: I'd put my uncle at 95%.

T: Let's see what other experiences could go on this scale.

(*Together, Joan and the therapist define and rate a variety of hate experiences, from an obscene phone call at 35% to the bar assault at 100%.*)

T: Now that we've filled in more of this scale, where would you put Patty when she was angry at you?

J: I guess at about 45% on this scale. But I felt so bad.

T: Sure you did. It's not easy to have someone we love get so angry at us. But it seems important to put her anger in perspective in terms of whether and how much she hated you. What difference does it make to you if her hate level was 45% instead of 100%, as you thought?

J: I feel a little better. And I think maybe I didn't need to break up with her. That makes me feel weird.

In this session, the therapist replaces the Thought Record with a scale as an instrument to test beliefs. For clients who adamantly reject data gathered on a Thought Record, the scale provides a more flexible and user-friendly tool for investigating beliefs. This is because a scale allows for incremental belief shifts in response to data rather than searching for a new perspective in response to cumulative data, as on the Thought Record. Eventually Joan will benefit from using Thought Records, but first she needs to develop some basic flexibility in thinking. She needs to learn that her thoughts are not facts but perceptions.

TREATING AXIS II DISORDERS

In addition to treating Axis I problems such as depression and anxiety, *Mind Over Mood* can be used to treat Axis II disorders directly.

When maladaptive schemas are weakened and alternative, more adaptive schemas are developed personality disorders can be successfully treated. Treatment is successful when a client meeting full diagnostic criteria for a personality disorder no longer meets the diagnostic criteria by the end of treatment. Case studies attest to the potential efficacy of cognitive therapy for personality disorders based on schema change and development of alternative behavioral coping patterns (Beck et al., 1990). Some suggestions follow for using the treatment manual to assist this therapy approach.

Changing Core Schemas

For a detailed description of clinical methods used to change core schemas, see Padesky (1994a). This section highlights the use of the treatment manual to facilitate schema change. Summaries of methods used to identify and change core schemas are provided along with clinical illustrations.

Identifying Core Schemas

Chapter 9 of *Mind Over Mood* includes the primary cognitive tools necessary to identify and change negative schemas. Worksheets 9.1, 9.2, 9.3, and 9.4 ask questions to help clients identify negative core schemas about the self, others, and the world. It is important to help clients identify all three types of schemas because these cognitive domains interact. As a cluster, these three types of schemas help explain emotional, behavioral, and motivational responses better than any single schema. For example, two people may have the self-schema "I am weak." If the first person has the other-schema "Others will hurt you if they get the chance," he or she will try to hide this weakness for self-protection and may adopt an avoidant style. If the second person has the other-schema "Someone is always weaker than I and deserves to be taken," she or he will be on the alert for weaker people and try to take advantage of them, adopting an antisocial pattern of coping.

Once maladaptive schemas have been identified and stated in the client's own words, alternative schemas can be identified. Pages 143–152 in Chapter 9 of *Mind Over Mood* can be used to help a client identify more adaptive schemas and state them in the client's own words. The process of identifying current schemas and desired new schemas can take several weeks, during which changes often occur in the words or concepts used to label the schemas. It is especially important to identify an alternative, more adaptive schema that has a desirable meaning for the client because this new schema forms the foundation of schema change processes. The following dialogue between Gary and his therapist illustrates the search for an alternative schema.

T: Last week we talked about your negative core belief "I'm no good" and came up with the alternative belief, "I'm good enough." I asked you to think this week about the phrase, "I'm good enough," to see if it captures how you'd like to see yourself. Did you do that?

G: Yes. It would be nice to see myself that way. But I don't think it's quite right.

T: What's not right?

G: When I think, "I'm no good," it's not just me I'm thinking about. It's how other people see me.

T: So is it more like "Others see I'm no good"?

G: No. That's not it, either. I think it's "I'll be punished for my faults."

T: I see. That is a different meaning. What would be the alternative to that? How would you like it to be?

G: Safe. (*Pauses.*) I'm safe even if others see my faults. (*Shoulders relax, eyes moisten.*)

T: How does it feel to say that?

G: Good. Scary. Relief, if I could ever believe that.

T: Let's write this down, "I'm safe even if others see my faults," and you can think about this idea this week and see if it seems to capture how you'd like things to be in your life.

In this interchange, the therapist listens carefully and asks questions that help Gary articulate a nuance to his negative schema that was out of his awareness before he tried to construct an alternative core belief. Note that Gary had moderately strong affect when the new alternative belief was stated. Schemas are closely tied to affect and clients usually show some emotion when an old or new schema is named for the first time. Gary's disbelief that the new schema could be true is also a characteristic response to an alternative, more adaptive schema.

Gary identified a schema somewhat different in form from the schema statements provided in Chapter 9 of the manual, "I am_____," "Others are_____," "The world is _____." His negative schema combines aspects of both self ("I have faults") and others ("Others will punish me"). It is important to help clients state the negative and alternative schemas in the form most meaningful to them and not force them to conform to the manual's template. Schemas take many shapes including images. For example, one woman had a pictorial schema of a small critical gnome sitting on her shoulder and worked to develop an alternative, more adaptive image. Once old and new schema are identified, clients can use the exercises in Chapter 9 of *Mind Over Mood* to actively work on schema change by weakening their conviction that the old schema is true and strengthening their confidence in the alternative belief they have constructed.

Schema Change Processes

A change in core beliefs requires simultaneous efforts to weaken old schemas and strengthen new ones. The manual includes worksheets to guide the client to use three primary schema change processes: continuum practice, core belief records, and historical tests of schemas. The following therapy excerpts show how Gary used each of these methods to weaken his schema "I'll be punished for my faults" and build confidence in the alternative schema "I'm safe even if others see my faults."

Continuum Methods

T: How does that new alternative belief, "I'm safe even if others see my faults," fit for you this week?

G: That seems like what I'd like. But the more I think about it, the more I'm sure it's impossible.

T: What makes it seem impossible to you?

G: I've never been safe. At work, at home, people clobber me if I screw up.

T: Let's make a safety scale. (*Draws a line and labels endpoints 0% and 100%.*) Here's 0% safety and here's 100% safety. At the top we'll write, "How safe I am when others see my faults." Where do you generally think of yourself on this scale?

G: At 0%.

T: Put an "X" at 0%, Gary, and note that that is where you see yourself.

(*Gary puts an "X" at 0% and writes "Me."*)

T: Now, let's make a list of times others have seen your faults.

G: Last week at work when I couldn't figure out the sales tax when my calculator broke. Let's see, I promised my son I'd fix his toy but I was too tired and didn't do it. That's all I can think of right now.

T: Any times you can think of when I've seen your faults?

G: When I first came here, I'd agree to do some work in the book and then I wouldn't do it.

T: So it sounds like when you say, "my faults," you mean mistakes you make or times you don't follow through on what you promise, or things you don't know how to do.

G: Yeah, that's right.

T: What do you mean by "safe"?

G: Safe from being hurt.

T: Physically hurt? Or emotionally hurt?

G: Both. When I was a kid my dad would beat me up pretty bad when I screwed up. But I feel just as bad if someone makes fun of me or calls me dumb.

T: Has that happened to you, too?

G: Yeah. In school, and sometimes at work my boss will get mad and call me a "dumb _____."

T: So let's write on this scale what safety means for you. At 0% let's write what no safety would mean. For example, you might get beat up until you're almost dead.

G: Yes. Beat up real bad or attacked and stood up in front of the group to be made fun of. (*Writes these ideas below 0% on the scale.*)

T: What would 100% safety look like?

G: I'm not sure.

T: Well, if 0% is being beaten within an inch of your life, I guess 100% safety would be feeling protected from physical harm.

G: Like having a bodyguard.

T: Yes. What would be the safest you could imagine?

G: Protected by a safety shield so no one could touch me.

T: OK. Write that under 100% safe. (*Pauses while Gary writes.*) Now, what about 100% safe from public shame or criticism? What would that look like?

G: If people were patient and encouraging me, instead of making fun of me.

T: Write that under 100% safe. (*Pause while Gary writes*) On this scale we are making, what would 50% safe look like? Something halfway between these endpoints.

G: Physically, I guess being shoved but not hurt. And I guess someone being critical or upset with me one-on-one, not in front of a group.

T: Write those down under the midpoint of the continuum, which we'll label 50%. Now, let's mark on this scale these three experiences you gave me where others saw your faults. First, you couldn't figure the sales tax at work when your calculator broke. Where would you put your safety then?

G: Hmmm. I guess about 25%. My boss made fun of me but only one other person was there and he didn't beat me up or anything.

T: Put an "X" there and label it so you know what the "X" means. (*Pauses.*) And how about when you didn't fix your son's toy?

G: I guess about 80%. He was disappointed but he wasn't mad at me.

T: Put an "X" there and label it. (*Pause*) How about in here when you didn't do what you said you would in the book?

G: Well, you didn't beat me up. (*Laughs.*)

T: Did you expect me to?

G: I sort of did.

T: And what did happen?

G: You asked me questions and were nice about it. And you helped me be not so afraid of screwing up.

T: So where would that go on this scale?

G: I think 90% safe.

T: Write that down. (*Pauses.*) Now we've got four "X's" on this scale, one for where you see yourself (0%) when others see your faults and three for recent events (25%, 80%, 90%). What do you notice when you look at this scale and these marks?

G: Where I see myself is different from what has happened lately.

T: Good point. What if we put some of your childhood events here, like that time your dad beat you up for making a mistake?

G: That would be 0%.

T: So, do you think as a kid you lived in 0% safety more often?

G: Not all the time. But I never knew when my dad would blow up.

T: So, seeing yourself as 0% safe might have been a good thing to do as a kid. I mean, it might have been better to assume you were never safe and be careful since you never knew when your dad would blow up.

G: Yeah. I think that's true.

T: How about today? Do you think it's still better to assume you're never safe?

G: (*Pauses*) No, I guess not. It looks from this line here that I may be safer than I think.

T: And what would be the advantage for you in thinking of yourself as being safer? Why not still think of yourself as only 0% safe?

G: Well . . . I could be more relaxed if I felt safer. And maybe I'd face up to people more.

T: And how do you think that would help you?

G: If I acted stronger, my boss might back off. He doesn't give Pete as hard a time as he gives me.

T: That's an interesting idea. It might be good to find out if your boss would back off if you acted stronger. We could practice in here how you might do that. First, though, maybe it would be helpful to keep track on this scale how safe you are this week when others see your faults. It might help to find out more about when you are safe and when you are not. What do you think?

G: That makes sense.

In this session, Gary's therapist uses a scale and guided discovery to begin to weaken Gary's conviction that he is 0% safe and also to introduce the concept of safety in the face of having faults. The first step of changing schemas is usually clarification of schema concepts. The therapist in the case example asks Gary to specify what he means by "faults" and "safety," then introduces a scale that provides a visual summary of Gary's experiences to assess whether they support or contradict his schema.

A scale or continuum is most therapeutic when it is constructed and its data evaluated for the new schema rather than the old. A small shift that strengthens the new schema is usually more hopeful for the client than a small shift that weakens the old schema. Consider the difference Gary would probably feel if he moved to "It's 90% true that I'll be punished for my mistakes" versus "I'm 10% safe when others see my faults."

Once a scale is constructed for the new schema, the therapist helps Gary qualitatively define the endpoints and midpoint. It is important to help the client label the endpoints in extreme terms so that the entirety of human experience is accounted for on the scale. On their own, clients sometimes define the endpoints in more moderate terms, which weakens the value of the scale to measure change. For example, if Gary had defined 0% safe as "Someone is displeased with me," then there would be little room for variability across the scale and his father's beatings would end up equivalent to his boss's reprimands and his son's disappointment.

Once the endpoints are defined, the therapist asks Gary to place recent experiences on the scale. She then asks Gary to compare his schema-driven perception that he is 0% safe when faults are revealed to his actual experience. Note that the therapist does not focus single-mindedly on disproving the schema. She links Gary's schema to early developmental experiences and empathically notes the adaptive value of his schema growing up with a physically abusive father. Once the origins and occasional adaptiveness of the old schema are validated, the therapist asks Gary to consider if this schema is always adaptive in his current circumstances.

Construction and use of scales in session helps clients begin to use scales to evaluate their schemas outside session using *Mind Over Mood* Worksheets 9.7 and 9.8. These worksheets direct the client to rate the new schema rather than the old. Worksheets in the manual thus support therapeutic emphasis on strengthening new beliefs rather than simply weakening old ones.

Continuum work is central to schema change because schemas are dichotomous. Use of a continuum or scale helps the client learn to evaluate experiences in more graduated terms. Small changes in belief that might be missed on a Thought Record are captured on a continuum. Since schemas change gradually in response to an accumulation of experiences, clients usually need to use scales and other schema change methods for six months or longer before a new schema is fully developed.

Core Belief Records. Since schemas shape our perceptions, they make it difficult for us to perceive information inconsistent with our current views. Therefore, clients do not see and remember experiences that could support alternative, more adaptive schemas. Sometimes called a positive data log (Padesky, 1994a), the Core Belief Record presented in Worksheet 9.6 of *Mind Over Mood* is designed to help clients notice and record experiences that support new schemas. Figure 7.1 shows an example of Worksheet 9.6 as Gary completed it.

WORKSHEET 9.6. Core Belief Record: Recording Evidence That Supports an Alternative Core Belief

New Core Belief: *I'm safe even if others see my faults.*

Evidence or experiences that support the new belief:

1. *Jim helped me when I couldn't get the bolt off.*

2. *Sally was nice when I told her about my bad day.*

3. *My therapist didn't get mad at me for forgetting my manual.*

4. *Bob just laughed when I couldn't understand the tax form. He*

   said he didn't understand it either.

5. *I stumbled reading a story and my son didn't seem to mind.*

6. *Sally and I made up after I got mad and we had a fight.*

7. _____

8. _____

9. _____

10. _____

---

11. _____

12. _____

13. _____

14. _____

15. _____

16. _____

17. _____

18. _____

19. _____

20. _____

21. _____

22. _____

23. _____

24. _____

25. _____

FIGURE 7.1. Gary's Core Belief Record.

Notice that Core Belief Records are designed to collect very small daily experiences. Ideally, the client finds two or three examples per day to write in the log. The difficulty in this seemingly simple task is that clients cannot easily perceive data that contradicts schemas. Until the new schema is strengthened, the client does not have the lens to bring this data into focus. At the same time, the data are necessary to construct the new schema. The therapist must therefore be alert to small experiences that support a new schema and help make the client aware of them so that the client can begin noting and recording them. Gary and his therapist illustrate this process.

T: Did you add any items to your Core Belief Record this week?

G: No. I didn't have anything happen to write down.

T: So you didn't make any mistakes or show any faults this week? It must have been a pretty good week!

G: Not exactly. My truck broke down and I was late to work. And I was pretty depressed last weekend.

T: When those things happened, did you get punished by your boss or by other people around you?

G: No, not really.

T: What happened?

G: Well, I couldn't call in to work because I wasn't near a phone. But my boss was pretty understanding when he found out what happened. And Sally was pretty nice to me on the weekend. She tried to cheer me up and made an excuse for me so I didn't have to go to her mother's house.

T: So, if you look at your new schema, "I'm safe even if others see my faults," do you think either or both of these experiences might be small examples you could write on Worksheet 9.6 to show that this belief is sometimes true?

G: I guess so. I didn't think the events really related to being safe, though.

T: But if you were always punished for your faults, what would have happened these two times?

G: My boss could have given me a job warning and Sally could have gotten mad at me, I guess.

T: Yes, those would be punishments of a sort. But they didn't happen, did they?

G: No. Both of them were pretty good about my problems.

T: Do you think you could write these examples on your sheet for this week?

G: Yes. (*Writes them on his worksheet.*)

T: Maybe this week you could think each day what went wrong

and notice any way you messed up. Then, if you weren't punished for it, you could write it on the worksheet.

G: OK.

T: Let's write this plan down on the top of the worksheet page as a
reminder of what type of experience to write down.

Gary's therapist helps look for data that could have been recorded
on his log by asking about the type of experience Gary fears (making a mistake or having some sort of problem). The therapist assumes that Gary won't notice experiences that contradict his schema
and helps him to see that in fact in several instances during the
week when things went poorly, he wasn't punished. She asks Gary
to write the instances down immediately in his log and then helps
him construct a guideline to help him notice this type of experience in the future. The therapist has Gary write down the plan for
noticing data that support his new schema on the worksheet because the therapist knows that Gary will forget information related
to the new schema if he doesn't write it down. By the time Gary
can easily complete Worksheet 9.6 on a daily basis, his new schema
will be formed; once the new schema is in place, he will easily perceive supportive data.

Most clients need to keep a new Core Belief Record for about six
months before the new belief is firmly established and has credibility. Core Belief Records can be combined with continuum ratings to chart progress. For example, Gary kept weekly ratings of
his confidence in his new belief, "I'm safe even if others see my
faults" on Worksheet 9.7. Recall that he believed the new schema
0% when he first identified it. After one month of writing experiences on Worksheet 9.6, he believed the new core belief 10%. After
three months his confidence in his safety when faults were revealed
had increased to 30–40%. Six months after beginning the log, his belief in the new schema increased to 80% for most of his relationships.

Historical Test of Schema.   Worksheet 9.9 directs the client not only
to consider current data in evaluating the credibility of a new belief but also to look for historical evidence that the new belief applies to his or her life. Most schemas are formed in childhood.
Negative schemas skew our perceptions and recollections of our
whole life. Therefore, it can be worthwhile to look back in our history for data we may have missed or ignored because they didn't
fit our predominant schemas.

Just as clients often need the therapist's help in perceiving data to record on a new Core Belief Record, they often need help in identifying historical information that supports a new schema. A therapist can help a client recall information by considering what small bits of evidence might exist and asking questions to prompt memories of this information. It is helpful to ask about a variety of relationships and events as Gary's therapist demonstrates.

T: Today I'll show you how to use Worksheet 9.9 to look for evidence from your past that might support this new idea you're working on, "I am safe even if others see my faults." You've told me this was not true with your dad when you were growing up, but I wonder if maybe it was true with any other people.

G: What do you mean?

T: Well, to begin this worksheet, who were the other important people in your life, let's say between the time you were born and age two?

G: My mother and my brother.

T: Do you think you were safe with either of them as a baby?

G: As a baby, I think I was OK. My dad was overseas in the army then.

T: So what could you write for this age period? For example, if you tried to stand and you fell down, or if you cried or got sick, how do you think your mother and brother treated you?

G: I think they were nice to me. I could write that down for those years. (*Pauses while he does so.*)

T: What about ages two to four?

G: My dad came home then and things got crazy. Whenever he'd drink, he'd start hitting us. I remember one time I was sick and cried and he hit me over and over again. I bet I was only three.

T: So at home it wasn't very safe when dad was there.

G: No.

T: Were you ever anywhere other than home?

G: I went to my grandma and grandpa's house every summer for a few weeks.

T: What was it like there?

G: It was fun. They lived in an apartment in Chicago and my grandfather used to take me to the zoo and to the train yards. We did lots of neat things.

T: What happened if you were sick, or made a mistake, or showed a fault to your grandfather or grandmother?

G: They were always nice to me. One time I broke a dish and I started to cry because I thought I'd get a whipping, but my grandmother just hugged me and said it was all right. My grandfather helped me clean it up and he said, "Dishes aren't nearly as important as family."

T: Do you think these experiences fit more with your old core belief, "I'll be punished for my faults," or your new belief, "I'm safe even if others see my faults"?

G: With the new one.

T: Why don't you write these experiences on Worksheet 9.9 in the age 2–4 row?

Like Gary, even clients who had pretty horrendous childhood experiences can benefit from the historical test of schemas. It is not necessary to identify many experiences that support the new schema; even a few are meaningful to clients. Ideally, clients find one or two experiences per age period. If a client has no memory for certain age periods (as happens sometimes when children were badly abused or sexually molested), he or she can benefit from completing Worksheet 9.9 for whatever age periods are remembered.

Changing Problematic Behavior Patterns

Rather than judging behaviors characteristic of personality disorders as pathological, cognitive theory describes them as coping strategies that make sense in the context of core schemas. For example, guarded behavior by the paranoid client is adaptive, not pathological, in the context of the client's conviction that "others will always use or manipulate me if I'm not on my guard." Dependent behaviors are sensible coping strategies if a client believes "I am weak and vulnerable to be hurt. Others are stronger and can protect me."

Schema change is therefore accompanied by a therapeutic focus on learning and applying new behavioral responses. Chapter 8 of *Mind Over Mood* can be used to structure behavioral experiments designed to test old schemas and strengthen new ones. To evaluate his new schema, "I'm safe even if others see my faults," Gary had decided it would be good if he could directly express irritation in his relationship with Sally. Like many clients, Gary initially avoided behavioral experiments because of anxiety and a conviction that new behavior was dangerous. In the following session, Gary's therapist helps him overcome reluctance to complete the behavior experiment.

G: I didn't really say what I felt this week, like we talked about last week.

T: Did you forget to do this or decide not to?

G: I sort of decided not to.

T: What thoughts and feelings led to that decision?

G: Well, I felt scared. I thought it was too risky.

T: Give me an example of a time that felt too risky this week.

G: I was irritated with Sally on Saturday and I thought about telling her to back off and leave me alone for awhile. But I was afraid she'd get mad and it would be bad for me.

T: So what did you do?

G: I just worked on my car and turned up the radio so she couldn't talk to me.

T: And how did that work out for you?

G: I felt mad the whole time and kept yelling at her in my head. Later she came out to talk to me and I was sort of cold to her and she got mad.

T: So your old behavior didn't really protect you from Sally's anger?

G: No.

T: And yet saying what you felt in the beginning might have led to Sally getting angry, too.

G: I think so.

T: So maybe we need to plan one step beyond the new behavior.

G: What do you mean?

T: Do you think it would help if you had a plan for what to do if Sally gets mad when you tell her how you feel?

G: Yeah. I don't really do anything when she gets mad but maybe walk away or sometimes call her a name and then walk away.

T: I think Worksheet 8.1 in your manual would help. Let's find it and give it a try.

G: I've got it.

T: Let's write the thought we're testing at the top of the page.

G: (*Gary writes, "I'm safe even if I tell Sally what I feel."*)

T: In the columns you can write your experiment—that's what you're going to do—your prediction of what will happen, and possible problems that might come up. Let's do that for Saturday, just as an example.

G: So, for "Experiment" I could write, "Tell Sally to back off."

T: That's right. We can role-play later some different ways you could say that to her. And what was your prediction of what would happen if you did this experiment?

G: She'd get mad.

T: Anything else?

G: We'd have a big fight.

T: Anything else?

G: She'd want to split up.

T: Anything else?

G: No, that's enough!

T: OK, write those three predictions down: Sally will get mad, we'll have a big fight, she'll want to split up.

G: (*Writing*) This is where I get stuck. I don't know what to write where it says "Strategies to overcome these problems."

T: Let's talk about some strategies. I bet you'll have a tough time doing these experiments until you have a plan for how to handle problems that could come up as a result.

G: When she gets mad, I just freeze or else I explode.

T: Do you know anyone who handles it well when someone gets mad at them?

G: Actually, Sally does pretty good. She makes sales calls and customers get mad at her all the time.

T: What does Sally do to handle it when people get mad at her?

G: She listens and says, "I didn't mean to make you mad" and says "I understand" and says things like "This doesn't seem to be a good time to talk." I don't hear what they are saying

because she's on the phone, but that's what I hear her saying.

T: Do you think any of those comments would be helpful for you
to use if Sally gets mad at you?

G: Maybe. I could say, "Maybe we should talk later."

T: Let's write that down. That might be a useful strategy if your
fighting seems to be getting out of hand, but I'm not sure that's
the best place to start because it sounds a little like avoiding
talking to her about your feelings.

G: That's why it seems so good! (*Laughs.*) Maybe I could say I don't
want her to be mad.

T: OK. And what do you want from her?

G: I want her to listen and understand why I'm upset.

T: Do you think that would be a good thing to say to her? (*As Gary
nods.*) Why don't you write that down, too?

Gary and his therapist continued developing strategies for responding to Sally's anger, then worked on strategies for defusing a
big fight and on strategies for preventing a breakup. Gary developed several strategies to overcome each potential problem. After
completing the first four columns of worksheet 8.1, Gary and the
therapist role-played various problem situations and responses. At
first, Gary hesitated to respond to Sally (as role-played by the
therapist). The therapist coached Gary through a number of role-
plays until Gary felt pretty confident that he could be assertive in
the face of Sally's anger.

As the example illustrates, common reasons clients do not follow through on behavior change assignments include intense
emotions, hopelessness beliefs, negative predictions, and inadequate knowledge or skills to respond to problems that might interfere with behavior change. To successfully change maladaptive
behavior patterns, therapists help clients (1) identify roadblocks
to change, (2) devise strategies for overcoming them, and (3)
practice new strategies in the office until the client gains confidence and skill. Chapter 8 of the manual includes worksheets to
structure experiments and Action Plans, important behavioral
complements to cognitive strategies for changing schemas. Alternative schemas do not have credibility to clients until real-life
experiences support them.

TROUBLESHOOTING GUIDE

Crises That Sidetrack Progress

The therapy of some clients is characterized by frequent crises that interrupt skill building and interfere with goal attainment. For these clients, a treatment manual can be a crucial aid in keeping therapy focused. It is helpful if the therapist identifies common skill deficits that may predispose a client to crisis-level problems. For example, some clients become overwhelmed by emotion and act impulsively. Other clients lack assertion and become immersed in demanding relationships and overwhelming demands. Some clients function well during the daytime when activities and structure are plentiful and sink into depths of distress at night when few supports are available. A case example illustrates the use of *Mind Over Mood* with these clients.

Patty came to therapy reporting frequent bouts of depression and anxiety. Each week she arrived with new crises: relationship conflicts, walking off her job in tears, and financial problems resulting from impulse shopping. In addition to depression and anxiety diagnoses, her therapist diagnosed borderline personality disorder. Discussion with Patty revealed that each crisis was precipitated by intense affect followed by some impulsive action on her part intended to relieve the affect.

Patty's therapist focused initially on helping Patty identify and rate her moods (*Mind Over Mood*, Chapter 3). For each crisis, this was the first therapy task, followed by problem solving in session to resolve the crisis. Patty completed an assignment to identify and rate her moods three times per day during the initial weeks of therapy until she felt confident that she had this skill. Next, she and her therapist identified her "hot zone": at feeling ratings above 6 she was likely to act impulsively.

Next Patty and her therapist developed specific coping plans for medium and high (ratings above 6) levels of emotion. At medium levels of affect, she was encouraged to employ active coping to reduce the risk of entering her hot zone. Active coping involved (1) making an Action Plan (*Mind Over Mood*, Chapter 8), (2) as she learned the skills, identifying thoughts and completing Thought Records (Chapters 4–7) or (3) calling one of the people on a list of five supportive people she could count on in a crisis. She was encouraged to rotate the friends she called so that none of them would feel overburdened.

Even with this plan in place, Patty often ended up in her hot zone because she frequently reached an emotional 9 or 10 rating within moments of a distressing event, so she and her therapist worked on a plan for high-affect crisis coping. The plan entailed a timeout to calm herself and make choices before acting. In-session role-plays and problem solving helped Patty learn socially acceptable ways to temporarily leave a situation (e.g., excusing herself to think it over or attend to a prior commitment with a promise to resolve the issue at some specified future time).

During her timeout period, Patty used a variety of coping methods, depending on the emotions she experienced. Usually she felt terrified or enraged, so she practiced a variety of methods to calm down when feeling these emotions. She and her therapist made a "coping grid" (Padesky, 1994b) for each emotion, a 2-by-2 chart

Feeling: Enraged	
Day	**Night**
Alone Write out my feelings	Play calm music
Play calm music	Write in my journal
Run or bicycle	Read my Thought Records
Hold an ice cube until it	from similar situations
melts	Make hot tea; sip it slowly
Slow breathing	Stretching exercises
Cook	Listen to my therapy tape
Call Randy or Pat	Take a hot bath
With Say I need to make a	Get to a safe place
Others phone call	Avoid alcohol
Slow breathing	Slow breathing
Walk away if I can	Speak slowly
Ask for understanding	Focus on a friendly person
Take a bathroom break	Leave if no one feels safe
Speak slowly	Call Marilyn if I need
Focus on a friendly person	company

FIGURE 7.2. Patty's coping grid.

labeled "Day" and "Night" across the top and "Alone" and "With Others" down the side. In each cell of this grid she marked coping behaviors for the target emotion. Figure 7.2 shows Patty's coping grid for the emotion "Enraged."

Patty used the strategies in her coping grid until she could rate her emotions less than 6. Sometimes a few minutes of coping were sufficient, although several hours of coping practice were often required to reduce the intensity of her emotions. Once she attained a more moderate level of emotion, she was able to use *Mind Over Mood* to understand the situation better and respond to it using Thought Records (Chapters 4–7) and Action Plans (Chapter 8) if appropriate.

Identification of Patty's skill deficits for tolerating intense moods led to initial therapy goals of learning to identify moods and manage them with behavioral coping strategies. Clients who experience intense, overwhelming affect find behavioral strategies easier to learn and practice than cognitive ones early in therapy. Once Patty learned to replace impulsive behavior with other strategies, she was more capable of using the therapy manual to understand her emotional reactions and develop problem-solving skills. The therapy manual provided structure to her learning at each step of therapy.

Objections to a Structured Therapy Approach

Occasionally clients with personality disorders object to structured learning, written exercises, or some other aspect of using the treatment manual. Avoidance, suspicion, or anger could underlie client objections; case examples illustrating these reactions and therapeutic guidelines for responding to them were presented early in this chapter of the clinician's guide. In this section, we suggest troubleshooting guidelines to help clients who object to therapy structure but do not fit into the categories described earlier in the chapter.

A negative client response to therapy should be heard and carefully evaluated. Identify client affective and cognitive reactions and find out as much as possible about what aspects of the therapy and your therapeutic style trigger them. It is important not to assume that the problem resides in the client. Clients with personality disorders can be expected to respond more strongly to interpersonal aspects of therapy than other clients; strong responses do not mean that these reactions are unwarranted.

As an example, one client felt hurt when his therapist enthusiastically pointed out a worksheet that could help him identify thoughts related to feelings of rejection. The client angrily confronted the therapist, saying she was more eager to teach him how to use the worksheet than to listen to his feelings in a situation that had been very painful for him. Fortunately, the therapist was open to client feedback. She recognized that the client was accurate in his perception. In her enthusiasm to introduce Thought Records, she had neglected to empathically listen to her client. It would have been better for her to introduce the Thought Record after she listened to and summarized his concerns.

Clients who object to written exercises and other aspects of therapy structure often do so because they fear that structure will reduce the quality of the therapy relationship. If this concern is raised, collaboratively examine the relationship and your therapeutic style. Are you practicing cognitive therapy in an overly prescriptive manner, referring constantly to worksheets and exercises even when rapport is absent? The therapy relationship is especially central with clients with personality disorders. It is important to maintain good eye contact, express caring and interest in the client, and listen well with empathic comments. Clients react to written work best within a strong collaborative relationship. With many clients with personality disorders, this relationship needs to be reestablished in each session.

Therapists also err if they push therapy too quickly. Session pacing is important. Do not ask six rapid-fire questions. Instead, ask a question, make a reflective response, pause, ask another question, and make frequent summaries of what you hear to allow the client a chance to check the accuracy of your perceptions. Another common therapist error is asking questions in a challenging fashion (e.g., "Are your sure that's what he meant?"), which contributes to a client perception that the therapist distrusts client perceptions. It is much better to pursue guided discovery in a manner that respects client perceptions and at the same time encourages the client to consider alternatives:

C: He just about came out and said he thought I was a loser.

T: What was it about how he said it that gave you that impression?

C: He had a superior look on his face. And he didn't even look me in the eye when he said he wasn't interested.

T: I can see how that could convey the idea he thought you were a loser. Did he say or do anything that implied anything different?

C: No.

T: Tell me a little more about his style. Did he talk to you any differently than he talks to other people?

C (*pausing*): I'm not sure. He does seem to cut off other people pretty quickly.

T: Why do you think he does that?

C: I'm not sure. Sometimes I think he's not very comfortable since he's younger than the rest of us.

In this excerpt, the therapist is trying to determine if the client can be sure that his friend meant to say he was a loser. However, instead of directly challenging the client's conclusion, the therapist helps the client identify the data that led to the conclusion and then begins to look for data that might support alternative interpretations. The Thought Records in the treatment manual follow the same pattern: Clients are asked to write down "Evidence that Supports the Hot Thought" before considering "Evidence that Does not Support the Hot Thought." If therapists are intent on disproving distressing thoughts, the therapy process loses credibility; clients perceive that the therapist is discounting negative aspects of their life experience. Good cognitive therapy helps clients face both positive and negative aspects of their experiences.

Sometimes the structure of the therapy needs to be modified to support a client's learning style. Clients who become anxious with math may wish to use color rating scales or use pictures or a pie chart instead of a scale. Schemas also may lead to modifications in the structured aspects of therapy. For example, some clients with histrionic personality disorder find the exercises more interesting when they relabel them with more dramatic titles in their own words. For example, a client might rename the Thought Record "Moods, Mind Games, and My Answer!"

One client had the schema "I must perform perfectly or others will leave me." She worked so diligently to please her therapist that each exercise in the treatment manual took her one hour or more to complete, and even then she was anxious that it would not be good enough. To reduce the schema-driven anxiety related to structured therapy worksheets, the therapist asked her to leave each exercise partially incomplete and to intentionally cross out words on the worksheets to make them appear less perfect. This adjustment, while initially distressing, helped the client reduce her perfectionism and provided early behavioral experiments to support schema change.

Remember that the importance of structure in cognitive therapy is to enhance learning. If structure impedes learning, it should be modified. Therapists who are ambivalent themselves about structure sometimes eliminate structure if clients object to structure. This is usually a therapeutic error. Sometimes clients who have the most difficulty following a structured therapy approach are those who benefit most by learning to be more structured. Therefore, it is best to reduce or modify therapy structure rather than eliminate it. Most clients readily follow a structured therapy approach if the therapist listens to concerns about structure, clearly explains the advantages of the structure employed, and is willing to modify the structure in response to client concerns.

If client and therapist cannot reach agreement on the degree and type of structure that is therapeutically ideal, behavioral experiments can be used to evaluate each person's ideas. One session or a portion of each session can be conducted following the structural desires of the client (e.g., "No questions, no writing, I just talk") and another session or portion can follow the therapist's proposal (e.g., "I ask occasional questions and help you write summaries or diagrams to connect your emotions and thoughts"). Following the experiment, both therapist and client can describe what was helpful and not helpful about each approach. The two then search for a compromise therapy plan that incorporates the useful aspects of both structures (e.g., "I will signal you when I want to talk without questions or summaries. After five minutes of listening, you will summarize what you've heard. If we decide there is an important idea, we will write it down").

Conviction That Change Is Impossible

It is not unusual for clients with personality disorders to be convinced that they cannot change. Psychotherapists often share this opinion, indeed part of the definition of personality disorders is that they are "enduring patterns" of "inner experience and behavior" that are "inflexible" and "stable." (APA, 1994, p. 629) It is countertherapeutic for therapists to believe that a client cannot change because therapist expectation influences therapist behavior and therapy outcome. For example, a therapist who believes that a client cannot change may initiate a therapy plan for change but accept stagnation in progress as inevitable. In contrast, a therapist who believes change is possible actively problem solves when progress is stalled and makes adjustments in the therapeutic plan until change is achieved. It is helpful for therapists to ask themselves, "What would I do with a client who did not have a personality disorder diagnosis if I ran into this difficulty?" Or, "If change is inevitable, how can I alter the treatment plan to help it come more quickly?"

A first step, therefore, with clients who believe they cannot change is to find out if this belief has been reinforced by other mental health professionals with whom they have worked, including yourself. Many clients have been told by well-meaning professionals that their problems will be lifelong. If this is the case, begin by discussing your own beliefs about change and possible differences in the current treatment approach from past ones.

C: What's the use? I can't change. I was born this way and I'll always be this way.

T: Where have you gotten the idea you can't change?

C: It's obvious. I never have changed even though I've been in therapy for years.

T: What have past therapists told you about change?

C: Some tried to be nice about it, like you. But the more I think about it, Dr. Grayson was right.

T: What did Dr. Grayson say?

C: He said that some people are born with musical talent and some people aren't. And some people are born with the skills to have an easy time in relationships and other people aren't. He was very kind about it. He said I was doing my best if I learned to be less angry with people, but I couldn't expect to get along like others all the time.

T: So he said you could change a little but not a lot.

C: Yeah. And I have changed a little. So there's no point in hitting my head against the wall. It just won't get any better than this.

T: This is an important idea for us to discuss. How do you suppose Dr. Grayson knew how much you could change?

C: I guess from his training and experience.

T: When did you see him?

C: A few years ago.

T: Did you and he do the same sort of therapy we are doing together?

C: No, it was different. We mostly talked about things. He didn't give me specific things to try during the week.

T: As you probably know from your experience, there are different therapy approaches. Depending on the approaches used, therapists work with problems in different ways.

C: Yes.

T: In addition, we learn more each year and new therapy methods are developed and tested, so some things we thought were hard to change five years ago are easier to change now. For example, in the 1970's I did not have many ideas about how to help people with panic disorder, and now I find I can help panic disorder really easily.

C: So are you saying Dr. Grayson was wrong?

T: I'm not sure. Dr. Grayson may have been right for that time and the approach he was using.

C: But you think I can change?

T: Yes, I do. And I think we can come up with things for you to learn and try in between appointments that will help you change.

C: But what if I can't change? What if it's not you or your approach, what if it's me?

T: Would you like to change?

C: Of course. I'm miserable.

T: In my experience, if people want to change, we can usually figure out a way, even if it means changing our approach a number of times until we figure out what helps.

C: I'm sorry, but I'm not sure I believe that.

T: You don't have to believe it. The good thing about change is that it is possible even if you don't believe in it. Many of the people I work with don't believe they can change. All I ask is that you try out the things we think might help and give me honest feedback on how these things make it better or worse for you so that we can keep adjusting our plan.

C: I can do that.

T: Would you like to give it a try then?

C: Yes.

T: And I don't want you to just go along with me on faith without change happening. So let's be sure to set some goals and review our progress every few weeks to make sure we are getting somewhere.

In this session, the therapist confronts central beliefs about change. It is important to openly discuss change beliefs because hopelessness can undermine change efforts. For example, this client believes additional change is not possible. With this belief, the client is likely to interpret setbacks as representative of life's reality for her. She will view any progress as a fortunate but temporary fluke. The client's attitudes predispose her to accept setbacks and mistrust progress.

The therapist does not insist the client share his confidence that change is possible. Beliefs about change are often schema driven, and therefore they are not easily changed. Rather than engage in a battle to convince the client that change is possible, the therapist introduces the possibility of change with a plausible rationale. The client is asked not to believe in this plan but to participate in it, give the therapist regular feedback, and help evaluate progress.

Also, it is helpful not to denigrate previous therapists or question their therapy methods unless the prior therapist has been clearly unethical or unprofessional (e.g., sexually involved with the client). Even previous therapists you may think are inept may have been helpful to a client in many ways, and there is no therapeutic benefit in undermining a client's positive reactions to a previous therapist. An emphasis on differences among therapy approaches and new developments in psychotherapy can foster client hope without detracting from other therapy experiences.

Once the client agrees to initiate a change plan and help evaluate its success, therapy can begin in earnest. It is important to set clear and attainable change goals. Large goals such as establishment of a close friendship should be broken into smaller initial goals such as maintaining a pleasant conversation with someone. Chapter 3 of this guide thoroughly discusses goal-setting procedures. Progress toward goals should be measured on a continuum to avoid all-or-nothing thinking. A continuum allows the client to acknowledge both progress and setbacks. A dichotomous question such as "Have you successfully changed?" often elicits a negative answer because the client with negative schemas regarding change perceives setbacks more readily than progress.

With clients for whom very slow progress and frequent setbacks are likely, it is important to set very small, observable goals. In addition, metaphors for change can often help reduce discouragement in both client and therapist. One particularly helpful metaphor is that of a spiral staircase. One client with borderline personality disorder was particularly despondent following a suicide attempt and hospitalization, her fourth hospitalization in a year. Note how the spiral staircase metaphor helped transform her perspective on this setback.

C: Here I am again. I'm so disgusted with myself and you must be, too. You may as well give up. I'm never going to change.

T: (*After a long pause*) I wonder how we'd know if you changed.

C: What?

T: Have you ever been on a spiral staircase?

C: Yes.

T: When you round the first bend and look out, what do you see?

C: Oh, a tree and a building.

T: Now, if you keep going up the staircase and you round the next bend, what do you see?

C: The same tree and building.

T: Does it look exactly the same?

C: Yes.

T: Are you sure? Would there be any change at all in what you see, no matter how small?

C: Well, maybe a slight difference in perspective. You might see a little higher up the tree or into a window on the building.

T: So the view would look essentially the same, with a slight difference in perspective.

C: Yes.

T: Do you think you're making progress when you climb a spiral staircase?

C: I see what you're getting at.

T: What's that?

C: That you can seem to be in the same place sometimes even if you are making progress.

T: I think so. And maybe the only way to know if you are stuck or making progress is to see if there is any change in perspective.

(Pauses). You and I have been in this hospital a number of times now. Is there is any difference between this hospitalization and the past ones to show us that we might be making progress?

C: Well, in the past I always yelled and attacked you when you first showed up. I didn't do that today.

T: Why not?

C: I guess I believe now that you put me here because you care, not because you hate me.

T: Do you think that's progress?

C: Yes.

T: Any other changes in perspective, even small ones, that show we are moving forward?

The spiral staircase metaphor and other metaphors of change can help both client and therapist maintain hope and enthusiasm for therapy progress even when patterns that characterize personality disorders are repeated over and over again. With consistent efforts to change schemas and behavioral experiments to change behavioral patterns, clients with personality disorders can change to the degree that they no longer meet criteria for a personality disorder. In the absence of long-term therapy to accomplish this goal, briefer therapy can help them learn skills to overcome Axis I difficulties. And no matter what the length of therapy, use of a treatment manual fosters skill attainment and consolidation of learning to help maintain more changes over time.

RECOMMENDED READINGS

Beck, A.T., Freeman, A., Pretzer, J., Davis, D.D., Fleming, B., Ottaviani, R., Beck, J., Simon, K., Padesky, C., Meyer, J., & Trexler, L. (1990). *Cognitive therapy of personality disorders*. New York: Guilford Press.

Freeman, A., Pretzer, J., Fleming, B., & Simon, K. (1990). *Clinical applications of cognitive therapy*. New York: Plenum Press.

Layden, M.A., Newman, C.F., Freeman, A., & Morse, S.B. (1993). *Cognitive therapy of borderline personality disorder*. Boston: Allyn and Bacon.

Linehan, M.M. (1993). *Cognitive-behavioral treatment of borderline personality disorder*. New York: Guilford Press.

Padesky, C.A. (1994). Schema change processes in cognitive therapy. *Clinical Psychology and Psychotherapy*, 1(5), 267–278.

Using MIND OVER MOOD in Brief Therapy

Often clients come to therapy for just a few sessions. Brief therapy may be a client's choice, mandated by a third-party payor, or a result of life circumstances such as plans to move out of the area. If the client has a single problem, a few therapy sessions may be sufficient to help. And even in a few sessions, *Mind Over Mood* can enhance the amount of learning and change that takes place in therapy. Clients can read chapters in the treatment manual and complete worksheets that reinforce the topics discussed in therapy sessions. The written records summarize learning for the client and identify areas in which the client is confused or "stuck." Written application of the principles discussed in therapy assure client and therapist that the client can use the ideas discussed in therapy to solve future problems independent of the therapist. The treatment manual also provides continued help for clients after brief therapy is completed. While it is ideal for someone to have a therapist's help in using *Mind Over Mood*, many people can use the book as a self-help manual when a therapist is not available.

Clients who come to brief therapy with multiple or complex problems present a much greater challenge for therapists. The remainder of this chapter can be considered a troubleshooting guide for conducting brief therapy with multiproblem clients. Consider the circumstances faced by three clients seeking help in brief therapy.

Carla arrives in tears at her first appointment. She has been depressed for five months. Yesterday her foreman told her the factory was closing at the end of the year. Two thousand people will be laid off in a county of 35,000 people. She and her husband have been quarreling for months and may get a divorce. Carla is worried about losing custody of the children if she has to move away to get a new job. She says she can't sleep or eat. Her insurance will pay for eight sessions of therapy.

Juan is nervous and fidgets during the first hour you meet with him. He reports panic attacks and waking up in the middle of the night in cold sweats. He says he has drunk heavily to "calm his nerves" for eight years, since he lost three buddies in a helicopter crash when he was in the Navy. Juan has not kept a job more than three months since leaving the service two years ago. He says his life looks empty and hopeless. The employee assistance counselor at his current company referred him to you for three sessions of crisis counseling.

Arlene reports a 22-year history of mood swings. Most of the time she is quite depressed but periodically she feels terrified or enraged. During these times she cuts herself with a razor blade. Sometimes she wanders the streets at night because she "feels so agitated," even in unsafe neighborhoods. She lives alone and would like to have friends but finds that people "can't be trusted." Public assistance funds will pay for two therapy sessions per month for Arlene up to a maximum of ten sessions per year.

These are typical examples of clients who need help in a time frame that is very brief relative to the number and complexity of problems they face. This chapter will show you how you can offer more therapeutic hours to clients such as Carla, Juan, and Arlene by using *Mind Over Mood* (1) as an integral part of brief therapy, (2) to bridge spaced therapy sessions, (3) to provide supplemental therapy, and (4) as a posttherapy guide. Which method you choose for a given client depends on the number of sessions available, client problems, client motivation, and client ability to use a treatment manual independent of a therapist. First, however, the importance of goal setting will be reviewed because setting clear goals quickly is the foundation for successful brief therapy.

GOAL SETTING IN BRIEF THERAPY

Goal setting is even more important in brief therapy than in longer therapy. With limited in-session hours available, it is critical for therapist and client to reach agreement as soon as possible regarding what client problems are most urgent and important to the client. All the client's problems cannot be solved in brief therapy. Brief therapy is of greatest assistance to clients like Carla, Juan, and Arlene if (a) one or two problems are solved and (b) the client learns skills for solving additional problems independently.

Chapter 3 of this guide describes strategies you can use to help clients set therapy goals. In brief therapy, it is usually best to start by addressing either the problem that is most urgent or a problem that underlies several difficulties. A good case conceptualization can help you and the client make these decisions in the absence of a crisis (Persons, 1989). To illustrate these two approaches to goal setting in brief therapy, consider Carla and Juan.

Goals Setting Based on Urgency

Carla arrives at her first therapy session in crisis. She is depressed, losing her job, and fearful of losing her husband and custody of her children. Eight therapy sessions will provide time to solve one or more of her problems and teach her a few skills to help solve the remaining problems. Which problem should be the focus of immediate help? Carla is unsure. She is tearful and distraught. Her therapist helps her set goals in the second half of the first therapy session.

T: Thank you for giving me this background on your problems. This is really a tough time for you and I'm glad you've come to get help. We have seven more meetings after today. We probably won't be able to completely solve all of these problems in seven meetings, but I'll work hard with you to solve as many of them as possible. Which one or two do you think would be most important to solve? (*Points to a list written in the first half hour, which reads, "depression, job search, marriage problems, child custody if we get a divorce, problems eating and sleeping."*)

C: (*Crying quietly*) I don't know. I just don't know.

T: Help me think this through, Carla. Some of these problems are happening right now and some are just possibilities. Maybe we could start with the problems that are certain. Which ones are those?

C (*looking at the list*): Well, I'm definitely depressed. I'm definitely losing my job. Our marriage is a mess. I'm not eating and sleeping.

T: So child custody is not an issue right now and might not be, if you don't get divorced.

C: Yeah. But I couldn't stand it if I lost my children.

T: I'm sure you'll do your best to prevent that from happening if you have to face that. For now, let's stick to your immediate problems. Which of the remaining problems are pressuring you the most right now?

C: They're all important. But I wake up worrying about my marriage. And I'm down all the time and that makes it hard to think.

T: So would it help if you were less depressed and we began to sort out the trouble in your marriage?

C: Oh, yes. But I don't think either is possible.

T: We'll see. We can always adjust our plan if we need to. Let me check on one thing first. How about your job? Why is that not such a big priority?

C: It will be nine more weeks until the plant closes. And we can make do with my unemployment check for awhile.

T: So you've got some time to solve that problem. (*Carla nods her head.*)

T: And if we helped your depression and marriage, you'd probably start eating and sleeping better.

C: Probably.

T: OK. I agree with you, then. The depression and your marriage look like your top problems. Now, which one of these do you think should be our number-one focus?

C: I don't know. What do you think?

T: I'm not sure either. Tell me, which problem started first?

C: Our marriage has been in trouble for a long time. I get so mad at Frank and he is totally fed up with me.

T: Do you think your depression is related to your marriage problems at all?

C: I don't think so. But I do get a real hopeless feeling when I think about what will happen if we divorce. It doesn't help.

T: It sounds as if we should work on both problems. Would you be willing to do some work in between our appointments to help your depression so we can spend most of our time here working on sorting things out with Frank?

C: I would, but I don't know what would help.

T: Before you leave today, I'll recommend a book and show you how to use it to help you with your depression. Each week when you come back I'll spend the first ten minutes or so reviewing your work in the book and answering questions you might have about your depression. Then the rest of the time we can work on your marriage. Does that sound OK to you?

(*Carla nods.*)

T: Do you think Frank would be willing to come with you to work on your marriage problems?

C: I think so, but he might want to talk with you on the phone first. He thinks a lot of therapists are screwy.

T: I'd be glad to talk with Frank on the phone. Let me show you this book, and then we'll decide how to set up the next appointment so you and Frank can come together. (Brings out *Mind Over Mood*, asks Carla to read the Prologue and Chapter 10, and shows her how to complete Worksheet 10.4 (Weekly Activity Record) to track her depression before the next appointment.)

In this session, the therapist helps Carla quickly decide which problems are most urgent for her to solve. Because Carla is in great distress and initially has difficulty prioritizing her problems, the therapist asks guiding questions to help her. When a client is in crisis and is overwhelmed by a number of problems, it is helpful to focus on solving the most immediate concerns. Other concerns (such as child custody in Carla's case) may disappear or become easier to solve once problems related to the immediate crisis are resolved.

Goal Setting Based on Case Conceptualization

Juan also arrives in therapy with a brief-therapy mandate (three sessions) for crisis counseling. Juan has several complex, interrelated problems, and three sessions will not provide enough time to improve his life considerably. Juan's therapist use's the time to conceptualize and define his problems in language Juan can understand to help him become more hopeful that his problems can be solved over time. If Juan is hopeful at the end of the three sessions, he may take the steps necessary to solve his problems.

At the end of the first appointment the therapist recommends Juan *Mind Over Mood* and asks him to read the Prologue and Chapter 1. He also asks Juan to write out the problems he experiences on Worksheet 1.1 (Understanding My Problems). In the second appointment, the therapist reviews Juan's worksheet, shown in Figure 8.1.

WORKSHEET 1.1: Understanding My Problems

Environmental changes/Life situations: Job changes, new apartment

Physical reactions: Cold sweats at night, tired

Moods: Panicky, nervous, irritated, angry

Behaviors: Quit jobs, drink too much

Thoughts: I hate my life. I'm a screw-up. Something bad is going to happen.

FIGURE 8.1. Juan's Worksheet.

T: You did a good job of filling out this worksheet, Juan. Did you learn anything from it?

J: Just that I've got a bunch of problems.

T: Yes, you do. Today I'm hoping we'll figure out a way of understanding how these problems fit together so we can help you feel better.

J: I'm afraid I'm just a hopeless case.

T: We'll see. One thing I notice is that under "Environmental changes/Life situations" you wrote about your job and apartment changes but nothing else.

J: That's about it.

T: Last week you talked to me about your Navy buddies dying in that helicopter crash eight years ago. I thought that was a pretty big stress for you.

J: But that was a long time ago. That shouldn't affect me now.

T: Let's talk about that. Do you remember Marissa in Chapter 1 of the manual? (*thumbs through* Mind Over Mood *to find the list of Marissa's problems on page 8*.) Under "Environmental changes/ Life situations" she wrote about being molested as a child and her abusive husbands even though those things happened a number of years ago. Do you think she shouldn't be affected by those things?

J: I can see how she would be. I saw a TV movie about this woman who was bothered for 40 years about what her dad did to her.

T: What happened in that movie?

J: Well, she faced her family and told everyone. It was real rough for her, but then she kind of accepted it.

T: So something bad from the past caused her lots of trouble until she faced it, talked about it, and came to some peace in herself about it?

J: That's right.

T: Do you think it might be like that for you with the helicopter crash?

J: What do you mean?

T: Are you at peace about the helicopter crash or does it still come up in your mind and bother you—like when you wake up in the middle of the night in cold sweats?

J: I guess it still bothers me some.

T: Why don't you write the helicopter crash on your worksheet, and then let's see if any of your other problems might be connected to that experience.

J: OK. (*Writes "helicopter crash" on Worksheet 1.1 in the "Environmental changes/Life situations" section.*)

T: Do you see any connection between the helicopter crash and any of these other problems?

J: Well, my drinking. And some of my nervous times.

T: How do you think your drinking is connected to that accident?

In the second session, the therapist helps Juan see the connection between the helicopter crash he witnessed in which his friends were killed and some of his current problems. The therapist is conceptualizing Juan's problems as the result of posttraumatic stress disorder (PTSD). Since Juan's heavy drinking, nervousness, and panic attacks all began soon after he saw his friends die in the helicopter crash, the therapist thinks these problems are secondary to PTSD. If so, therapy will be more helpful to Juan if the focus is on this trauma. However, Juan must agree with this conceptualization for therapy to proceed; it will not proceed if he objects to a focus on the meaning of a past event when he has so much current distress.

When Juan dismisses the helicopter crash as too far in the past to be influencing for his current problems, the therapist draws his attention to Marissa in Chapter 1 of *Mind Over Mood* because traumatic past events affected her current life. The therapist avoids direct disagreement with Juan's belief that past events are unimportant. Instead, the therapist applies the clinical observation that people who discount information about themselves often are more objective in evaluating comparable information about other people.

Juan is able to see the relevance of past traumas for Marissa. Her story reminds him of a television movie about incest. After the discussion about Marissa, Juan can see how his own traumas are comparable to Marissa's. The therapist uses relevant information from the television movie to help Juan conceptualize the link between his own trauma and his current problems. Stages of trauma recovery that Juan recalls from the television movie can then be used to introduce Juan to a rationale for the treatment steps that might be necessary to solve his problems.

Importance of Skill Building

No matter how brief the therapy, skill building is a desirable therapy goal en-route to solving problems. The skill learned may be methods of conceptualizing problems, identifying and testing thoughts related to a given problem area, or developing Action Plans to solve problems.

Each chapter of *Mind Over Mood* teaches at least one skill. Assignment of one or more chapters from the treatment manual highlights the skills a client is learning. While a client's immediate distress may lead to a narrow focus of attention on one problem, the treatment manual is a reminder that skills that solve one problem can be applied to others. Familiarity with *Mind Over Mood* gained in therapy can lead to independent client use of the manual to help resolve ongoing and future problems. For example, if Juan is intrigued by what he learns discussing Worksheet 1.1 with his therapist, he may read more chapters in the manual after his three consultation sessions. The treatment manual teaches many of the skills Juan can use to overcome his anxiety, panic, hopelessness, drinking problems and erratic job performance; clients described in *Mind Over Mood* experience problems that are like Juan's (Linda experiences panic attacks, Vic is a recovering alcoholic, Marissa expresses hopelessness and has survived many traumas).

USING *MIND OVER MOOD* AS AN INTEGRAL PART OF BRIEF THERAPY

Carla's therapist demonstrates how integrating *Mind Over Mood* with brief therapy can nearly double the impact of eight therapy sessions. Recall that Carla chose two major problems as her brief therapy focus: depression and her troubled marriage. *Mind Over Mood* allows the therapist to devote careful attention to both problems simultaneously.

Carla is willing to use *Mind Over Mood* to learn the methods of cognitive therapy for depression between therapy appointments. The therapist recognizes that Carla will need some help overcoming a depressive (i.e., self-critical, globally negative, and hopeless) response to her life difficulties. At the same time, Carla is used to working hard (she works full-time and raises children) and seems committed to feeling better. The therapist therefore judges that about ten minutes of each session will be sufficient to clarify questions and review Carla's progress using the worksheets in *Mind Over Mood* to overcome her depression.

Of course, this initial plan can be modified if Carla has more difficulty than anticipated learning the necessary skills. However, as long as she is successful in using the treatment manual for her depression, the major portion of each therapy session can be devoted to helping Carla and Frank improve their relationship and resolve conflicts. In fact, *Mind Over Mood* also can be used in the couple's therapy to teach Carla and Frank to identify the hot thoughts behind their mutual anger (Chapter 5) and to use Action Plans and behavioral experiments to structure changes designed to improve their relationship (Chapter 8).

As Carla's therapy illustrates, whenever a client has two or more major problems, *Mind Over Mood* can be used to guide client improvement in one area while therapy sessions focus on another. Independent use of the manual should be reserved for problems that are simplest to resolve and that can be solved largely through the client's individual efforts. Even though depression can be a complex problem for some clients to resolve, Carla's therapist thinks that for Carla it will be easier to handle on her own than the marital problem. Therapist time should be devoted to more complex problems, with a portion of each session devoted to review of the client's work in the manual. This review alerts the therapist to unanticipated difficulties or client misunderstandings that require greater therapist intervention.

Therapy is additionally enhanced if the therapist points out to the client similarities in the skills used to solve problems. For example, in couple's therapy, Carla and Frank can learn to identify and test their perceptions before exploding in anger—the same skills Carla practices as she completes Thought Records to reduce her depression. Carla is so encouraged that the skills she is learning in session and on her own can be used to solve diverse problems that she decides to use Thought Records to help her during the job search process.

USING *MIND OVER MOOD* AS A BRIDGE FOR SPACED THERAPY SESSIONS

Mind Over Mood can function as a bridge to guide client learning between widely spaced therapy sessions. With a treatment manual as a guide, highly skilled and motivated clients can tolerate many weeks between therapy appointments. Clients who have difficulty maintaining momentum for change or who lack necessary knowledge and skills often cannot benefit from widely spaced therapy sessions unless they have written material to help cement learning.

Arlene is an example of a client who lacks skills and internal resources for coping. Arlene experiences chronic problems with depression, terror, rage, and self-mutilation. She engages in high-risk behaviors, such as wandering dangerous streets at night, and she is socially isolated. Arlene needs therapeutic help, but her public assistance funds limit her to ten sessions of therapy per year, no more often than twice per month. Given the likelihood that Arlene will experience emotional crises several times per week, she needs to learn better skills for handling her emotions than cutting herself and wandering the streets. She would also benefit from learning when and how to trust people.

Mind Over Mood provides Arlene with a new way to learn how to cope. Arlene benefits greatly from early chapters in the treatment manual. Frequently overwhelmed by vague yet intense feelings of distress, Arlene at first does not know how to distinguish among her emotions. Although difficult for her to learn, she finds it useful to distinguish between the situation, her emotional reactions, thoughts, and behaviors. Chapter 3 becomes a well-worn chapter because she struggles to name specific emotions, saying instead, "I feel evil." The therapist helps Arlene see the benefit in naming emotions by constructing coping grids with her, which summarize what she can do to cope with various emotions such as "sad," "furious," and "frightened." For an example of this therapy method, see the coping grid shown in Figure 7.2 on page 155 of this guide.

The ten therapy sessions in the first year focus exclusively on helping Arlene learn the skills in Chapters 1 through 4 of the treatment manual and on constructing coping plans (Chapter 8) for various problem situations (both emotional and interpersonal). Arlene experiences a few successes using coping plans, such as avoiding a conflict with a confrontive neighbor. She remembers to use her coping grids occasionally when she is sad or frightened, although when angry, she is still most likely to resort to cutting herself.

The treatment manual serves as a bridge to Arlene's second year of therapy. In therapy, the manual provides a focus for discussions with her therapist. Using the book lowers the necessity for intense therapist–client interaction, which had raised her anxiety intolerably in previous therapy relationships. Between her first and second 10-session therapy years, *Mind Over Mood* provides a link to the therapist that helps maintain Arlene's willingness to return to therapy. At the end of the first year's sessions, Arlene and the therapist write out a plan for continued use of the manual to guide practice of the skills she has begun to learn.

As Arlene's therapy illustrates, *Mind Over Mood* can be used to consolidate skills as well as expand the learning that occurs in brief therapy. If a client can attend only a few sessions of therapy, the sessions can be spaced several weeks apart using the manual to structure client learning between appointments. If a client is in crisis, the therapist can meet with the client three or four weeks in a row and then allow several weeks between the final appointments to allow time for the client to apply skills learned. Between the final appointments, *Mind Over Mood* can guide client coping and problem resolution. Remaining therapy appointments can be used to work on problems and roadblocks to change that the client cannot solve using the treatment manual alone.

USING *MIND OVER MOOD* AS A SUPPLEMENT TO BRIEF THERAPY

Sometimes *Mind Over Mood* is best used as a supplement to brief therapy. Juan was sent to therapy by his employee assistance counselor for three sessions of crisis counseling. The therapist spent the first two sessions helping Juan see the link between his various problems and the trauma he had experienced years earlier when he saw several of his Navy friends killed in a helicopter crash. In the third session, Juan's therapist reviewed the various options available to help him overcome his posttraumatic stress reactions.

In addition to recommending direct therapy for PTSD and alcoholism at a local VA hospital, the therapist suggested that Juan use *Mind Over Mood* on his own to learn more about anxiety, panic, and other emotional reactions. The therapist wrote down specific chapters for Juan to read to learn skills for solving each of his problems. The therapist's suggestions followed the treatment protocols outlined in Chapters 4 through 6 in this guide.

USING *MIND OVER MOOD* AS A POSTTHERAPY GUIDE

For brief therapy clients, *Mind Over Mood* provides a helpful reference and posttherapy guide for continued learning. Although the treatment manual does not address every problem for which people seek therapy, it does teach "common denominator" skills that can help clients solve a wide range of problems. It helps clients understand their problems, identify feelings, identify the thoughts connected to feelings, gather data that does and does not support their thinking, generate alternative views of problem situations, develop Action Plans and coping strategies, and evaluate core beliefs.

Clients can be directed to use *Mind Over Mood* after therapy in different ways depending on skill strengths and deficits. Clients who have greater awareness of emotions and flexibility in their thinking often can use the treatment manual independently with ease. Clients who have particular skill deficits can use particular chapters of *Mind Over Mood* as remediation. Among the clients described in this chapter, Carla came to therapy with the greatest number of psychological skills, Juan was intermediate in skill level, and Arlene had the greatest skill deficits.

As a result of her high skill level, Carla was able to use *Mind Over Mood* as a comprehensive posttherapy treatment program. Her depression had improved considerably during brief therapy when she used the treatment manual with limited therapist assistance. During therapy, she was able to use *Mind Over Mood* to identify and test thoughts that maintained her depression and also those that fueled her anger with Frank. Following therapy, Carla continued to use the treatment manual to work on her depression. After five months, her depression completely remitted. She continued to use various chapters in the book to solve other problems that emerged in her life.

Carla also independently used Chapter 9 of *Mind Over Mood* to identify the core belief "I'm no good," which she recognized sustained a number of interpersonal patterns that led to conflict with and resentment toward Frank. She used the worksheets in that chapter to increase her awareness of this belief and replace it with the belief "I'm good enough."

Juan continued to use *Mind Over Mood* to learn more about the thoughts and feelings that sustained his anxiety. He found the book particularly helpful for learning to identify emotional reactions to situations. Juan also successfully identified key thoughts that fueled his anxiety, including frequent images of the helicopter crash in which his friends were killed. His group treatment program at the VA hospital was partially cognitive–behavioral, so Juan felt the manual had given him a head start in the program.

Arlene used *Mind Over Mood* in a variety of ways over her years of treatment. In the first year she used it to help identify feelings and separate feelings from behaviors, thoughts, situations, and physical experiences. As she learned to identify and test her thoughts in the second cycle of therapy sessions, Arlene used the Helpful Hints boxes in Chapters 5 through 7 to help identify and evaluate her reactions to people and situations in her life. These skills helped attenuate her moods somewhat.

Arlene's functioning fluctuated depending on the number and intensity of stressors in her life. *Mind Over Mood* was most helpful to her when she was functioning relatively well and she felt that the skills she learned helped her function better more often. During periods of poor emotional functioning, Arlene often forgot or chose not to use the book. She would occasionally sink into vegetative depression or enter periods of enraged hostility directed at herself or others.

When Arlene was attending therapy during these times, her therapist was able to help her achieve emotional balance within a few days. If her ten sessions for the year were over, Arlene sometimes had "evil days" for weeks at a time. After noting this pattern in her second year, she and her therapist decided that her third year of therapy would consist of crisis-only sessions to reduce the length of these periods of low functioning. Arlene was instructed to try to use *Mind Over Mood* as a first resort in times of trouble. If she was not able to use the manual to achieve emotional stability within a few days, she would call her therapist for an appointment.

ADDITIONAL TREATMENT SERVICES

Many clients attending brief therapy can be helped by a variety of services in addition to a treatment manual. For example, Carla might have benefitted from antidepressant medication in addition to *Mind Over Mood*. However, as mentioned in Chapter 4 of this guide, the skills taught in the treatment manual are linked to lower relapse rates for depression, so antidepressant medication alone may not be the ideal treatment for depression. In fact, physicians offering medication alone as treatment for depression, anxiety, and other mood-related problems could add depth and breadth to their treatment by using *Mind Over Mood* in their protocol.

Juan benefitted from a variety of services for his problems, including the VA hospital group treatment program for alcoholism and PTSD. Other clients with substance abuse problems might be referred to Alcoholics Anonymous, Rational Recovery, S.M.A.R.T

Recovery or other treatment programs. Arlene benefitted from a number of additional services including medication, social service assistance with job training, and a community treatment program for the chronically mentally ill. Many clients can also benefit from involvement in community activities that are not related directly to mental health, such as churches, volunteer programs, activity groups, classes, senior citizen centers, and special interest programs (e.g., an art program, a community softball league, or a cultural festival).

For some clients in brief therapy, cognitive therapy via *Mind Over Mood* may be the sole intervention. For other clients, the treatment manual may be only a portion of the treatment plan. The advantage of using *Mind Over Mood* in brief therapy with multiproblem clients is that the skills the manual teaches apply to many dimensions of life. In all likelihood, the skills and strategies taught in this treatment manual will offer effective interventions for many of the difficulties experienced by a client. *Mind Over Mood* provides a toolbox clients can use to solve problems not fully addressed in a brief course of therapy.

RECOMMENDED READING

Dattilio, F.M., & Freeman, A. (Eds.). (1994). *Cognitive-behavioral strategies in crisis intervention.* New York: Guilford Press.

Using MIND OVER MOOD with Groups

Outpatient cognitive therapy groups offer cost-effective, clinically efficient help for many problems including depression, anxiety, couples problems, stress, pain, substance abuse, and eating disorders. The same active, directive, and problem-focused approaches used in individual cognitive therapy are used with groups. This chapter describes how *Mind Over Mood* can help structure and guide cognitive therapy in a group setting.

Prior to establishing a group, several decisions need to be made. Will the group be time-limited or open-ended? Will it be guided by one therapist or cotherapists? Will the group have a homogenous or heterogeneous population with regard to diagnosis, gender, age, or other variables? Both time-limited and open-ended groups can be effective, although session content are somewhat different in each, as described later in this chapter. Therapists new to a cognitive therapy approach, group therapy, or *Mind Over Mood* often find it helpful to work with a cotherapist until familiarity with this approach and skill in implementing it are achieved.

Diagnostically homogenous groups have the advantage of simplicity; a single treatment protocol can be helpful for all group members. It can be difficult, however, to find a group of clients with similar clinical profiles ready to begin a group at the same time. But since cognitive therapy skills are effective for many different problems, heterogeneous groups are also beneficial. While diagnostically mixed groups do not pose a problem for clients, they do require therapists to have more extensive knowledge and the flexibility to respond to both individual and group needs.

The desirability of group homogeneity for gender, age, ethnicity, or other client variables depends on group and client goals. Clients sometimes find it socially enjoyable or feel more at ease meeting in groups with high similarity. On the other hand, diverse group demographics help group members learn that human problems are more similar than different across age, gender, economic, educational, and ethnic boundaries. For example, members of a depression group were startled to discover that an 80-year-old man and a 22-year-old woman had the same types of negative thoughts and often stated them in the same words. The cognitive similarity of two seemingly different people taught a powerful lesson on the connection between thoughts and depression.

Once decisions on group format are made, the group can be formed. Before the first group meeting, it is recommended that each prospective member attend a pregroup individual screening interview to assess the client's problems, motivations, and expectations. Individual sessions allow the therapist the opportunity to meet group members, help define individual goals, identify special needs, and screen out those clients who do not fit the preestablished guidelines for the group.

PRINCIPLES OF GROUP COGNITIVE THERAPY

Group cognitive therapy progresses similarly to individual cognitive therapy. The members first become socialized to therapy and then progressively learn a hierarchy of skills. Just as the therapy relationship is important in individual therapy, the group relationship is important in group therapy. Therefore, group therapists strive to facilitate positive group cohesion and interactions, encouraging group members to be mutually collaborative and supportive of individual members' change efforts. If group conflict occurs, the therapist encourages clear communication to resolve disputes.

Similar to individual cognitive therapy, group sessions are structured by the use of agendas, encapsulated summaries, and written or verbal skills practice. Collaboration and guided discovery are central therapy processes; the therapist follows the guidelines in Chapter 1 of this guide. Clients practice new skills and test beliefs inside and outside the sessions. As in individual therapy, the group therapist can follow the chapters in *Mind Over Mood* sequentially to structure and organize each group session.

Agenda Setting. At the beginning of each cognitive therapy group session, the therapist(s) and group members set an agenda or list of topics they wish to discuss. Therapist suggestions for the agenda usually include leftover topics from the previous meeting, review of the past week's homework, and a new teaching/learning topic. Group members often want help with individual problems, raise questions, or offer updates to the group on their progress.

If many agenda items are suggested, the therapist can search for themes that consolidate two or more items into one. For example, if two clients want to talk about panic attacks they had during the week, both may do so as part of one agenda item. If another group member has a question regarding identification of automatic thoughts, it too can be folded into the agenda item on panic attacks. The agenda item might be to use the first three columns of a Thought Record (which include identification of automatic thoughts) to understand the panic experiences.

Collaboration. Recall that collaboration in individual cognitive therapy refers to the therapist and client working together as a team to solve a mutually agreed-on problem. The same spirit is fostered in group cognitive therapy. All group members work together on each agenda item. Group members learn to ask each other questions to gather empirical evidence and test automatic thoughts or beliefs. When one group member is testing a belief, other group members offer suggestions or ask questions to help bring alternative data to light.

Encapsulated Summaries. In individual cognitive therapy, clients provide encapsulated summaries of what has been discussed in order to consolidate learning before moving to another agenda item. In group cognitive therapy, encapsulated summaries are provided by the client(s) working on the agenda item or by another group member. Summaries can be written on a board and/or group members can write them in their treatment manuals for future reference. Additionally, the therapist can refer group members to the relevant page or chapter in the treatment manual for further reading, clarification, and practice of learning points discussed in group.

Client Feedback. Therapists are encouraged to ask each group member for feedback on the helpfulness of the group, pacing, the therapist's style, and other variables affecting client progress and learning. This information allows the therapist to make adjustments and also to gauge the progress of each group member.

Homework. Homework assignments are an integral part of individual and group cognitive therapy. Ideally, homework assignments are collaboratively constructed following the guidelines in Chapter 1 of this guide. It is a challenge to find adequate time to follow the important cognitive therapy principles for homework assignments described on pages 24–27 of this guide for each group member. Therefore, the therapist should alert group members to the principles he or she wishes to follow in assignment of learning exercises. For example, group members can be asked to collaborate in development of assignments that are relevant, simple, and practical, and that build skills and hold importance for them. Clients and therapist can mutually decide on homework assignments based on these principles, what was learned in the group, individual goals, and the clients' level of skill development. In more advanced groups, clients can help each other devise individual homework assignments. When clarification of learning or skill development is needed, chapters or exercises in *Mind Over Mood* may be appropriate homework assignments.

MIND OVER MOOD COGNITIVE THERAPY GROUPS

Mind Over Mood can help focus group sessions and build client skills when group members bring the treatment manual to each group to complete exercises, share homework assignments, take notes, and chart progress. For group therapy based on the manual, one or more chapters are assigned each week either sequentially as they appear in the manual or in an order specified by a treatment protocol (Chapters 4 through 6 of the guide). When group members report difficulty with a particular skill, extra group time is spent clarifying and practicing that skill.

An example of an eight-session group oriented to teaching clients the skills necessary to complete Thought Records, behavioral experiments, and Action Plans follows. Each 90-minute group session and pregroup and postgroup individual sessions are described with recommended assignments from the treatment manual. Adapting the eight sessions for a twelve-session group is also explained, and the four extra sessions for a twelve-session group are described.

SUGGESTED AGENDA

> **Pregroup Individual Session**
>
> • Assess and diagnose client.
> • Set client goals.
> • Orient client to the *Mind Over Mood* group.
> • Introduce *Mind Over Mood*—chapter topics, worksheets, mood inventories.
> • Assign homework: Consider the Prologue, and Chapters 1 and 2. Also consider Chapter 10, 11, or 12 and the *Mind Over Mood* Depression and Anxiety Inventories if relevant.

Pregroup Individual Session

Three important therapy goals are accomplished in the pregroup individual session: assessment and diagnosis, individual goal setting, and introduction to the group format. First the therapist interviews the client to assess current problems, past history, diagnoses, level of functioning, expectations, and other factors to determine suitability for the therapy group. Since group therapy does not permit much therapist time for individual members, clients with multiple acute crises or who are highly suicidal may be required to participate in individual therapy in lieu of or in addition to the group. The advantages and disadvantages of group therapy compared with other available treatments are discussed so that the client can use the meeting to assess whether the group format meets his or her needs.

If the client seems appropriate and chooses to participate in the group, individual expectations and therapy goals are discussed. Guidelines in Chapter 3 of this guide are followed to help the client set reasonable goals that can be accomplished during the time span of the group. Clients often need help setting specific goals.

Observable and measurable goals are set whenever possible so that the client can gauge his or her progress during group therapy.

If the therapist plans to use *Mind Over Mood* in the group, he or she can introduce the treatment manual to the client and explain how *Mind Over Mood* will be used to structure the group sessions. The first homework assignment can be assigned in the individual session to socialize the client from the beginning to active learning outside the group. Often the first homework assignment is to read the Prologue and first two chapters of the treatment manual. If the client has a predominant and troubling mood, part or all of Chapter 10, 11, or 12 also may be recommended. Clients who are depressed and/or anxious should complete the *Mind Over Mood* Depression and Anxiety Inventories and record baseline scores on the graphs in Worksheets 10.2 and 11.2. These initial readings and exercises in the manual help the client become familiar with cognitive therapy concepts that will be further explored in group sessions.

SUGGESTED AGENDA

> ## Group Session 1
>
> • Introduce members and review their goals (15 minutes).
> • Socialize members to group cognitive therapy (5 minutes).
> • Set session agenda (10 minutes).
> • Review Chapter 1: Understanding problems; five-component model with explanation and examples from group; Helpful Hints, on page 14 (20 minutes).
> • Review Chapter 2: Ask group for examples of the thought connection (15 minutes).
> • Introduce identification and rating of emotions (15 minutes).
> • Assign homework: Consider Chapters 3 and 4 (5 minutes).
> • Elicit and give feedback (5 minutes).

Group Session 1

In the first session it is important to introduce group members, develop group cohesion, socialize clients to therapy, and review initial reactions to and progress in the treatment manual. Then a new skill is introduced, homework is assigned, and the leader requests feedback. It is virtually impossible to accomplish all these goals in a 90-minute session unless the group leader is well-organized and willing to structure the session. A time allotment for each task is suggested in the Suggested Agenda. However, building group rapport and cohesion is the central task of the first session, so these times and even some of the learning tasks should be ignored if additional time is needed to create a collaborative atmosphere in the group.

Introduction of Group Members and Review of Goals

At the beginning of the first session, members are encouraged to introduce themselves and, if they are willing, to describe individual goals. By making their goals public, all members can support each other in individual goal attainment. A review of goals also provides the leader with feedback on how members understood the goals set in the individual pregroup screening session.

If group members read portions of Chapters 10 through 12 and completed the *Mind Over Mood* Depression or Anxiety Inventories, the opening minutes of the first session can be used to answer general questions about these chapters and to review scores recorded on Worksheets 10.2 and 11.2. Group leaders may wish to make copies of completed depression and anxiety inventories to review and track symptoms experienced over time. Group members who are depressed or anxious should be encouraged to complete the inventories weekly, record scores on the relevant worksheets, and bring worksheets to the session so that the group leader can review them.

Socialization to Group Cognitive Therapy

Following introductions and goal review, the leader describes the format, expectations, and guidelines for group cognitive therapy. When the structure and plan for each group session is stated, members know what to expect and can prepare to get the most out of each session. The following types of statements can be used, allowing ample opportunity for discussion of each point.

1. "Let me tell you some of the guidelines we find help group therapy go well. First, everything group members say should be kept confidential. That means you shouldn't tell your friends

or family what you hear about other group members. If you want to talk about yourself, that's OK. But each one of us has a right to privacy in what we tell others here. Do you agree with that? Any questions?"

2. "We will work as a group in these meetings. I will try to balance the time between different group members. This means you may sometimes not get to talk as much as you'd like. Or we may spend time on someone else's problem one week and address your concerns another. If you feel the time is unbalanced between group members, please bring this concern up in the session or during the feedback at the end of the session. The last five minutes of each session will be a feedback to review what was helpful to you and what you didn't like about the group."

3. "In fact, each session after today will follow a regular pattern. At the beginning of each meeting, we will plan our agenda for the session. Think about what you want to accomplish in each session and tell it to us at the beginning of the meeting. In the second part of each meeting, we'll review your learning experiences from the past week. Your individual experiences with learning assignments (reading, writing, or behavior experiments) will be discussed next. Then, I will introduce a new skill with group discussion and practice. Before the end of the session, each of you will receive a new learning assignment to bring you closer to your goals. We will end each session with five minutes of feedback. How does this plan sound to you? Any questions or changes you want to recommend?"

4. "In cognitive therapy, we think it's very important for you to learn methods for solving your own problems. Each week you will learn something new, and we want you to try out these ideas and see if they help you in your own life. Therefore, each week you will be asked to do some learning assignments such as reading, completing exercises in your treatment manual and trying out new behaviors or attitudes in your day-to-day life. This can be a fun part of the group learning process."

Setting the Session Agenda

Following discussion of the group format, members are encouraged to help construct the agenda for the first group. The group leader(s) describe the learning topics for this session and collaborate with group members to decide which member agenda items will be discussed to illustrate each topic.

Review of Initial Reactions and Progress in Mind Over Mood

Following orientation to the group, the first homework, assigned in the pregroup individual sessions, is discussed. The group reviews their reading and the written exercises they completed. The group leader can draw on the board the five-part model for understanding problems introduced in Chapter 1 and ask group members to describe the connections between these five parts of their experience that they noticed during the preceding week. A simple exercise such as this encourages group members to begin talking and participating in the group without high demands for self-revelation. The leader can check to see if all group members successfully completed Worksheet 1.1. Any questions about this worksheet can be answered by reviewing the Helpful Hints box on page 14 of *Mind Over Mood*.

If group members also completed Chapter 2 in the manual, the leader can ask them to summarize what they learned about the connection between thoughts and the other four parts of the model just discussed. Group members can offer personal examples of thought connections in their own lives and discuss their responses to Worksheet 2.1.

Introducing Emotion Identification and Rating

The group leader can introduce identification and rating of emotions in a variety of ways. Experiential exercises are always preferred over minilectures. The leader might ask group members to imagine themselves in a particular situation and then identify emotional reactions. Alternatively, group members can be asked to list all the emotion words they know to create a group mood list similar to that on page 27 of the treatment manual. A discussion can follow regarding how participants determine that they are feeling one mood rather than another.

Once the group demonstrates an ability to name moods, the leader initiates a discussion of mood ratings. Group members are asked to give examples of when a mild mood might be experienced relative to a strong mood and how the two feel differently. Individual variations in mood ratings are discussed, and group members are encouraged to develop scales that capture their own mood ranges rather than trying to identify a universal mood rating scale. In other words, a certain level of sadness may be rated 3 by one group member and 6 by another group member; each person has a unique range of mood experience.

Homework Assignment

A common assignment after the first session is Chapter 3 of the treatment manual, which provides information and practice regarding mood identification and rating. Clients can be encouraged to complete Worksheet 3.1, "Identifying Moods" and Worksheet 3.2, "Identifying and Rating Moods," relative to goal-related situations. For example, a client who has an individual goal of learning to speak in public could imagine herself in such a situation and identify and rate the moods that interfere with attaining her goal.

If the group leader thinks that the group will be able to complete Chapter 3 with some ease, Chapter 4 can be added to the assignment. This chapter introduces the Thought Record and the concept of distinguishing between situations, moods, and thoughts. (Concepts described in Chapter 4 are clarified in the second group meeting.)

Feedback

The final minutes of each session are spent eliciting feedback from group members. Members are encouraged to describe what was helpful about the meeting and what could be improved. A summary of individually significant learning points can be made. Discussion of pacing, time management, the group leader's demeanor, and other group process observations are encouraged. In order to reduce the likelihood of one group member attacking another during the feedback period, when there is no time to process interpersonal conflict, constructive criticism is emphasized: "This is the time to let me know if I am doing anything that makes the group a negative experience for you. I welcome all your feedback so I can help make this a good group experience for all of you. However, if you have feedback for other group members, give just the positive feedback now so they don't have to sit with negative feedback all week. If you have negative concerns about other group members, write them down and give them to me at the end of this session or raise them at the beginning of the next session so we can put them on our agenda for that meeting when we have time to talk them through."

The group leader can model constructive criticism by giving members positive feedback about their group participation that day. In addition, the group leader models openness to negative feedback by thanking participants for acknowledging aspects of the group they did not like. For example, if a group member complains that he or she did not get to talk enough about personal problems in the meeting, the leader might respond, "I'm glad you let me know you feel this way. That is one of the difficulties of group therapy. Sometimes it is difficult to meet individual needs. Did you feel I slighted you in favor of other group members today?"

In this response, the group leader welcomes negative feedback, restates the realistic limits of group therapy, and then asks for clarification to further explore the individual's complaint. If the individual and other group members felt that the leader was ignoring this member relative to others in the group, the leader would agree to pay careful attention to this pattern and discuss these concerns further in a subsequent meeting. If client complaints seem more idiosyncratic and perhaps schema driven, the group leader can respond following the principles outlined in Chapter 7 of this guide.

SUGGESTED AGENDA

> **Group Session 2**
>
> • Set session agenda (10 minutes).
> • Review homework: Chapter 3 and Worksheets 3.1 and 3.2 (15 minutes).
> • Review Chapter 4: Introduction, overview, and purpose of Thought Record (10 minutes).
> • Explain and clarify first three columns of Thought Record with examples from group (20 minutes).
> • Define and practice identification of automatic thoughts (20 minutes).
> • Assign homework: Consider Chapters 4 and 5 (10 minutes).
> • Elicit and give feedback (5 minutes).

Group Session 2

The second session begins with setting a session agenda and reviewing homework. It is important to review homework assignments near the beginning of each session to gauge skill development, correct misunderstandings, and emphasize the importance of completing between-session assignments. The new topics introduced in the second session are the Thought Record and identification of automatic thoughts.

The group leader focuses on skill building from the very beginning of each session, constantly assessing what skills group members have mastered and what individual questions and experiences can be used to build new skills for the entire group. The leader asks group members what items they want to put on the agenda. Clients may want to talk about a recent panic attack, suicide attempt, interpersonal conflict, and a host of other topics. The topics provide the focus for learning new cognitive skills. The group collaboratively chooses which topic(s) to explore in greater detail in the session. If clients want to discuss anxiety in the second session, the therapist can use that agenda item to demonstrate how to identify the automatic thoughts associated with anxiety.

The following vignette from a second group therapy session demonstrates how one group member's agenda item provided an opportunity for the group to see the connection between thoughts and feelings, learn to dissect an experience on a Thought Record, and practice identification of automatic thoughts:

THERAPIST: Lupe, your agenda item is next. You wanted to talk about being anxious about going to the mall.

LUPE: Yes, I really want to get over those feelings. I'm so full of fear.

THERAPIST: Let's talk about the time in the last week when you were most full of fear.

LUPE: Well, Saturday morning my neighbor asked me if I wanted to go to the mall with her in the afternoon. Just the thought of going made me so agitated, I couldn't stand it.

THERAPIST: I can hear the anxiety in your voice as you talk about it. On Saturday morning, at the moment that you were most nervous, what was going through your mind?

LUPE: I had an image in my head of being uncomfortable in the crowd at the mall. I pictured myself feeling disoriented and having difficulty telling anybody what I was going through. What if I fainted while I was there and no one knew how to help me? I decided to stay home. I told her I didn't feel well.

THERAPIST: You describe your mood as "full of fear." With 100 being the most fearful you have ever been and 1 being mildly fearful, how would you rate your fear when you had those thoughts?

LUPE: About 90.

(*At this point, the therapist goes to the board and draws the first three sections of a Thought Record.*)

THERAPIST: Lupe, this is a good example for showing how an experience can be understood on a Thought Record. (*Fills in first three columns, as shown in Figure 9.1.*) Does this accurately describe what you experienced on Saturday morning?

THOUGHT RECORD

1. Situation	2. Moods (Images)	3. Automatic Thoughts
Who? What? When? Where?	a. Specify b. Rate (0–100%).	a. What was going though your mind just before you started to feel this way? Any other thoughts? Images? b. Circle the hot thought.
Saturday morning. Neighbor asks me to go to mall with her later in day.	*Fear 90%*	*Image of myself being uncomfortable in the crowd at the mall.* *Picture of myself feeling disoriented and having difficulty telling anybody what I was going through.* *What if I faint?* *No one will know how to help me.*

FIGURE 9.1. Lupe's Thought Record.

LUPE: That's it in a nutshell.

THERAPIST: We will come back to this experience briefly and talk about alternatives to staying home. I want the group to recognize that any experience we have can be similarly examined on a Thought Record. By separating the situation, moods, and automatic thoughts, we can take a closer look at how our thoughts affect our moods and behavior. Who in the group wants to make a guess about how the images and thoughts going through Lupe's mind affected her mood and decision to stay home?

One of the goals of the second session is to articulate the connection between thoughts, mood, and behavior. The therapist may decide to ask other group members to describe their thoughts during periods of high emotion during the week. Underneath Lupe's Thought Record, the therapist can record on the board the experiences of other group members, thereby working with several clients simultaneously. Alternatively, all group members can be asked to fill out the first three columns of a Thought Record for one of their troubling events from the week either in the treatment manual on Worksheet 5.1 or on a separate sheet of paper.

Lupe's agenda item provides a springboard to teach all group members how to complete the first three columns of a Thought Record. The first three columns require skills group members have just learned (identification of situations, moods, and mood ratings) and new skills (identification of automatic thoughts). Now is a good time to introduce Chapter 5 of the treatment manual, which teaches how to identify automatic thoughts. In particular, clients can be advised to use the questions in the box at the top of page 51 of the treatment manual to help identify automatic thoughts in the coming week during situations with high mood ratings.

The stage and skill development of the group determine what is done with agenda items. In the second or third group meeting, problem situations are used as examples to identify automatic thoughts. In later sessions, the same situations provide opportunities to look for evidence that does or does not support hot thoughts and that can be used to construct alternative or balanced thoughts. In still more advanced sessions, the same agenda items are used to identify assumptions and core beliefs, to gather evidence for and against core beliefs, to help develop alternative assumptions and beliefs, and to devise behavioral experiments and Action Plans.

Group Session 3

- Set session agenda (10 minutes).
- Review homework: Chapter 5 (15 minutes).
- Explain and clarify identification of automatic thoughts and hot thoughts with examples from group members' worksheets 5.1, 5.2, and 5.3. (30 minutes).
- Define and practice gathering evidence for and against hot thoughts (20 minutes).
- Assign homework: Consider Chapter 6 and Worksheet 6.1 (10 minutes).
- Elicit and give feedback (5 minutes).

Group Session 3

The purpose of the third group session is to solidify clients' skill in completing the first three columns of the Thought Record and to introduce the next two columns—the evidence columns—so that clients can begin to evaluate their thoughts in problem situations. Any problems placed on the agenda can help group members consolidate their ability to identify automatic thoughts and hot thoughts. Lupe may have additional anxiety experiences to discuss, another client may want to talk about an argument with a friend, and a third may be struggling with severe depression. The group can use the questions in the box on page 51 of the manual to help each other identify automatic thoughts relevant to the problems being discussed. In this way, each group member is actively involved in the learning process for other members' agenda items.

Questions clients may have regarding hot thoughts are examined in this group session. It is important for clients to develop an ability to identify the hot thoughts that explain their emotional reactions because the remaining columns of the Thought Record pertain to these thoughts more than other automatic thoughts.

Group members can help each other decide if an identified automatic thought is a hot thought by discussing whether it best explains the mood experienced. For example, John may choose "It's not my fault" as the hot thought to explain his depressed mood, rated 80%, during an argument with his wife on Saturday. Group members can point out that this thought leads them to feel not depressed but relieved or even angry. If John has correctly identified his mood, group members might question him (using the questions in the box on page 51 of the client manual) to help identify his hot thought.

PEGGY: Maybe it wasn't your fault, John. But what was it about the argument that made you *depressed*?

JOHN: I don't know. It just seems we have this argument over and over again.

DAVID: What about that makes you depressed, John?

John: I think our marriage is doomed.

PEGGY: What would that mean to you, if it was?

JOHN: My whole life is ruined.

DAVID: If I thought that, I'd be depressed, too!

THERAPIST: Do you think this might be a hot thought, then?

GROUP: Yes!

THERAPIST: What do you think, John? Do you think "My whole life is ruined" is a hot thought that helps explain your depression on Saturday, or do you think there's a further thought to identify?

JOHN: Yes, that's what I thought. I still do think that and it makes me depressed.

THERAPIST: Maybe the group can help you with this thought today.

John's hot thought could be used as an example to teach the group how to look for evidence that does or does not support the thought (columns 4 and 5 of the Thought Record). It is important to emphasize the criteria for what constitutes evidence. Client assumptions and feelings are not evidence. Actual events and experiences are important evidence to write down. The group can refer to the Helpful Hints box on page 70 of the client treatment manual for questions they can ask John to help him find evidence that does not support his conclusion "My whole life is ruined."

The advantage of completing columns 4 and 5 of the Thought Record as a group is that most people evaluate other people's beliefs with greater flexibility than they do their own. Therefore, John gets help evaluating a belief that maintains his current depression, and other group members practice gathering evidence under fairly easy conditions for them. Following the group exercise helping John look for evidence to complete columns 4 and 5 of his Thought Record, the group summarizes what they learned and begins discussing the next week's learning assignments.

Most likely, Chapter 6 of *Mind Over Mood* (which discusses the evidence columns) is assigned, and group members are asked to complete Worksheet 6.1 (the first five columns of the Thought Record) for several situations. Group members may also self-assign additional learning assignments that are more action oriented. For example, John may talk to his wife about her hopes for solving their marriage problems or approach a friend to find out what support is available to him if his marriage does break up.

SUGGESTED AGENDA

> **Group Session 4**
>
> - Set session agenda (10 minutes).
> - Review homework: Chapter 6 and Worksheet 6.1 (30 minutes).
> - Explain and clarify gathering evidence for and against hot thoughts with examples from group members (30 minutes).
> - Assign Homework: Consider additional practice with Worksheet 6.1 (10 minutes).
> - Elicit and give feedback (10 minutes).

Group Session 4

The fourth session helps patients consolidate the skills necessary to complete the first five columns of a Thought Record. The group leader can peruse worksheets completed during the week and review important information as needed regarding mood identification and ratings, identification of automatic thoughts, selection of hot thought(s), and recording evidence that supports and does not support the hot thought selected for testing. Numerous examples should be used to illustrate the first five columns of the Thought Record. Group-assisted Thought Records often include interpersonal process data from the group, as illustrated by the following example in which David was assessing the thought "Others can't be trusted."

THERAPIST: David, where's the evidence that others can't be trusted?

DAVID: I've been divorced twice, my father abandoned me, and everyone I've ever been close to has hurt me. Give people enough time and they eventually will hurt you.

THERAPIST: David, how do you feel as you are talking?

DAVID: Sad. I'd rate it about 90%.

THERAPIST: That's interesting. David, is it OK with you if I write your thought on the board to use as an exercise?

DAVID: Why not?

(Therapist writes first four columns of David's Thought Record on the board, as shown in Figure 9.2)

THERAPIST: David, do you have any evidence that doesn't support these conclusions?

DAVID: No, not really.

THERAPIST: Who in the group has a suggestion for David on how to look for evidence that does not support his thought "Others can't be trusted"?

VICTORIA: David, have you ever trusted anyone who hasn't hurt you?

DAVID: No.

PAM: What about us, David? Do you trust people in the group?

DAVID: I guess . . . somewhat.

PAM: Has anyone in the group done anything untrustworthy?

DAVID: Not that I can think of—not yet, anyway.

THERAPIST: Have people done anything that suggests that you can trust them?

DAVID: Well, people seem concerned. No one has laughed at me. I guess no one has said anything that was hurtful.

THERAPIST: What does it mean that people in the group have not said or done anything hurtful?

DAVID: I know what you want me to say. You want me to say that I'm wrong and that people can be trusted.

THERAPIST: No, we're not trying to prove you wrong. You have some good evidence to support the idea that people can be hurtful. I'm just curious about what it means that no one in the group has said or done anything hurtful.

DAVID: Maybe they are different. Maybe this group is not the real world.

TOM: David, how much do you trust me?

DAVID: I trust you—I guess half and half—50%.

TOM: What could I do to get you to trust me even more?

DAVID: I guess that would take time.

In this interaction, group members ask questions to address the issue of trust in David's life and as it manifests in the group. The group addresses interpersonal processes simultaneous with building skills. The therapist may fill in column 5 of the Thought Record on the board with information taken from this interchange, (Figure 9.3).

THOUGHT RECORD

1. Situation	2. Moods	3. Automatic Thoughts (Images)	4. Evidence That Supports the Hot Thought	5. Evidence That Does Not Support the Hot Thought	6. Alternative/ Balanced Thoughts	7. Rate Moods Now
Who? What? When? Where?	**a.** What did you feel? **b.** Rate each mood (0–100%).	**a.** What was going though your mind just before you started to feel this way? Any other thoughts? Images? **b.** Circle the hot thought.			**a.** Write an alternative or balanced thought. **b.** Rate how much you believe in each alternative or balanced thought (0–100%).	Rerate moods listed in column 2 as well as any new moods (0–100%).
In group. Thursday, 7:30 p. m. Talking about trust.	*Sad 90%*	*Others can't be trusted. Give people enough time and eventually they will hurt you.*	*Divorced twice. My father abandoned me. Everyone I've ever been close to has hurt me.*			

FIGURE 9.2.   David's Thought Record, Columns 1–4.

THOUGHT RECORD

1. Situation	2. Moods	3. Automatic Thoughts (Images)	4. Evidence That Supports the Hot Thought	5. Evidence That Does Not Support the Hot Thought
Who? What? When? Where?	a. What did you feel? b. Rate each mood (0–100%).	a. What was going though your mind just before you started to feel this way? Any other thoughts? Images? b. Circle the hot thought.		
In group. Thursday, 7:30 p.m. Talking about trust	Sad 90%	Others can't be trusted. Give people enough time and eventually they will hurt you.	Divorced twice. My father abandoned me. Everyone I've been close to has hurt me.	I trust people in the group to some degree. No one in the group has done anything untrustworthy. No one has said anything hurtful. People seem concerned. No one in the group has laughed at me. I trust Tom 50%.

FIGURE 9.3. David's Thought Record, Columns 1–5.

Group members ask questions, comment on whether they view a piece of data as constituting genuine evidence, and provide their own data. Group members are usually quite engaged in helping each other complete Thought Records because it is often easier to see what is missing in the thinking of another person than it is to perceive shortcomings in one's own thinking. Group members often comment that they understand concepts discussed in the treatment manual more easily when helping other people; this is often the first step in learning to evaluate one's own firmly held beliefs.

The belief "Others can't be trusted" may be one of David's core beliefs. If so, homework exercises in Chapter 9 may be helpful for him. Specifically, Worksheet 9.5, the Core Belief Record, and the exercises designed to identify and strengthen alternative core beliefs (Worksheets 9.6, 9.7, 9.8, and 9.9) might help David learn to be more trusting over time. These worksheets and exercises can begin as an in-session group exercise and be continued between sessions.

SUGGESTED AGENDA

Group Session 5

- Set session agenda (10 minutes).
- Review progress toward individual goals (20 minutes).
- Review homework (20 minutes).
- Define alternative thinking with examples from group members (5 minutes).
- Define balanced thinking with examples from group members (5 minutes).
- Practice constructing alternative and balanced thoughts (Column 6) for partially completed (Columns 1–5) Thought Records (20 minutes).
- Assign homework: Consider Chapter 7 and Worksheets 7.1 and 7.2 (5 minutes).
- Elicit and give feedback (5 minutes).

Group Session 5

Although progress toward individual goals should be informally tracked by group members and the leader in each group session, the fifth session is a good point to evaluate whether individual cli-

ents are making reasonable progress. Clients who hoped for a reduction in depression or anxiety levels should be completing the
Mind Over Mood Depression and Anxiety Inventories (Worksheets
10.1 and 11.1) on a weekly basis and charting them on Worksheets
10.2 and 11.2. The graphs can be reviewed during this session. Many
clients, however, will not experience a significant drop in mood
scores until they learn the skills taught in the fifth and sixth sessions, so stable mood scores at this time are not necessarily a poor
prognostic indicator. Sharp increases in mood scores might indicate the need for adjunctive treatments, however. Individual,
couples, or family therapy; medication; or a new conceptualization
of client problems might be considered along with a review of the
client's skill in completing *Mind Over Mood* assignments.

Clients with goals for behavior change can assess if they are
making progress at a reasonable pace. Client avoidance can be addressed at this point by identifying the moods and automatic
thoughts that maintain it. Some clients may realize after a month
or so of effort that the original goals need to be changed or broken
into smaller steps. Any readjustment of goals can be written in the
treatment manual.

The major goal of the fifth group session is to introduce alternative or balanced thinking, column 6 of the Thought Record. It is
important for clients to understand that this column is derived from
the evidence gathered in columns 4 and 5. The Reminder Box on page
94 of the treatment manual summarizes for clients what constitutes
alternative or balanced thinking. The Helpful Hints box on page 95 of
Mind Over Mood summarizes questions clients can ask themselves to
complete column 6 of a Thought Record. These questions can be used
to help group members complete this column on some of the Thought
Records they worked on for homework the previous week.

Examples from group members can be completed so that everyone has at least one opportunity to practice alternative or balanced
thinking with group assistance. Once alternative or balanced
thoughts are written down, individual group members rate the
believability of the statements. It is not unusual for people to believe new perspectives on their situations only slightly. Group members can help each other decide whether the alternative and
balanced thoughts have poor believability because they are poorly
constructed or because the idea captured is simply new to a client,
even though other group members find it believable.

For example, continuing his Thought Record from the previous
session, David might write the alternative thought "Everybody is

trustworthy" in column 6 and rate its believability at 0%. This is not a good alternative belief because it does not account for the evidence in column 4 of his Thought Record (Figure 9.2). The group could point out to David that this statement has low believability to everyone. They might help David construct a more balanced thought, such as "Some people may be trustworthy. It takes time to build trust." This thought may only have 10% believability to David, but the rest of the group may agree that this thought fits the evidence of his life and seems highly believable to them.

Once group members have written a somewhat believable balanced or alternative thought in column 6 of a Thought Record, they rerate their mood in column 7. If a client thinks the alternative or balanced thought in column 6 is moderately to highly believable, he or she will probably experience a shift in mood. If there is no shift in mood, the Troubleshooting Guide on page 102 of *Mind Over Mood* can help determine the reason. Clients are ready to practice the complete Thought Record on their own following this session.

SUGGESTED AGENDA

Group Session 6

- Set session agenda (10 minutes).
- Review Chapter 7 and Worksheets 7.1 and 7.2 (35 minutes).
- Define and plan behavioral experiments (30 minutes).
- Assign homework: Consider first half of Chapter 8 and Worksheet 8.1 (10 minutes).
- Elicit and give feedback (5 minutes).

Group Session 6

In the sixth session there is further practice in completing Thought Records with focus on development of alternative and balanced thoughts for column 6. If clients do not experience mood change after completion of Thought Records, the Troubleshooting Guide on page 102 is reviewed. Often when alternative or balanced thoughts are only partially believable to the client, additional information is needed beyond that gathered on a Thought Record. It can be helpful for skeptical clients to conduct behavioral experiments to test an alternative thought.

Although behavioral experiments may have been recommended to individual clients in previous sessions, the sixth meeting is often a good time to discuss behavioral experiments in detail with the group as a whole. Group members can help each other plan interesting behavioral experiments to test alternative beliefs that are only partially credible or to try new behavioral coping strategies and evaluate their effectiveness. For example, Lupe might plan some experiments to face situations she has been avoiding; David might act more trusting in one or more situations and see what happens. Chapter 8 of *Mind Over Mood* describes how to plan these experiments, and Worksheet 8.1 can be used to structure client homework for the seventh session.

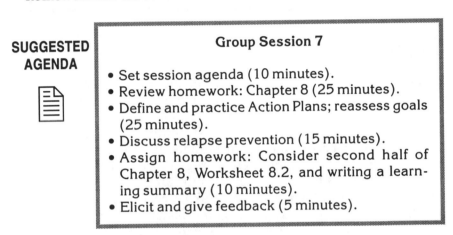

SUGGESTED AGENDA

Group Session 7

- Set session agenda (10 minutes).
- Review homework: Chapter 8 (25 minutes).
- Define and practice Action Plans; reassess goals (25 minutes).
- Discuss relapse prevention (15 minutes).
- Assign homework: Consider second half of Chapter 8, Worksheet 8.2, and writing a learning summary (10 minutes).
- Elicit and give feedback (5 minutes).

Group Session 7

In eight-session group therapy, the seventh session is used to begin preparing for group termination. Clients are encouraged to ask questions regarding problems they are still experiencing, reassess progress toward their goals, and make plans for continued progress after therapy is over. This is a good session in which to formally introduce Action Plans (*Mind Over Mood*, Worksheet 8.2) because Action Plans can be used to plot continued progress toward goal attainment after the group sessions end. In addition to other skills learned in therapy, Action Plans may also be part of a relapse prevention plan.

If the group is meeting longer than eight sessions, the seventh session can be used to review concepts and provide additional skills practice. Action Plans are introduced and group members are encouraged to use Worksheet 8.2 to plan concrete steps which will help achieve therapy goals.

SUGGESTED AGENDA

> ### Group Session 8
>
> • Set session agenda (10 minutes).
> • Review homework: Chapter 8 (30 minutes).
> • Review members' summaries of learning and goals met (30 minutes).
> • Discuss members' future plans, and allow time for goodbyes (20 minutes).

Group Session 8

If the eighth session is the final one for the group, members review and consolidate the gains they have made, discuss individual plans for continued learning and practice, say goodbye to each other, and arrange individual post-group sessions (see page 209). Group members should be encouraged to continue using the treatment manual to guide their change efforts in the months ahead. It is helpful for group members to summarize which skills are most helpful to them and which skills need additional practice. Members can discuss their ongoing plans for change and offer each other advice and encouragement for future individual efforts. Some group members may offer to continue meeting informally after the group has ended to support change efforts and help solve difficulties.

The group leader may also comment briefly on Chapter 9 of *Mind Over Mood*, offering brief guidelines for clients who plan to continue using the manual to identify and change core beliefs. Clients should be told that, although the other chapters of the book were mastered in a week or two, Chapter 9 exercises are designed to be completed over a number of months. Some group members may already have identified core beliefs during the eight group meetings; these can be written down at the top of Chapter 9 as a reminder.

If the group is meeting for twelve sessions, the leader can spend more time on earlier topics. One recommendation is to spend two weeks on identification of hot thoughts (session 3 for an eight-session group), a skill that often requires more than a week to master. In fact, a bit more time can be allowed at each stage to fully master skills. If group members are mastering skills at the pace of an eight-session group, additional meetings can teach more advanced skills.

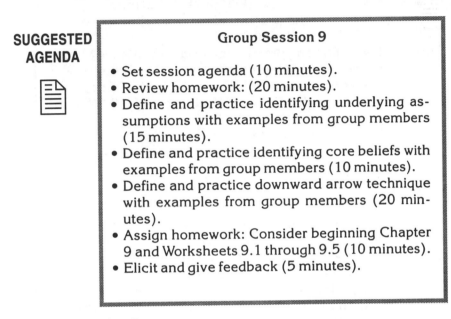

SUGGESTED AGENDA

Group Session 9

- Set session agenda (10 minutes).
- Review homework: (20 minutes).
- Define and practice identifying underlying assumptions with examples from group members (15 minutes).
- Define and practice identifying core beliefs with examples from group members (10 minutes).
- Define and practice downward arrow technique with examples from group members (20 minutes).
- Assign homework: Consider beginning Chapter 9 and Worksheets 9.1 through 9.5 (10 minutes).
- Elicit and give feedback (5 minutes).

Group Session 9

The ninth session may be used to explain and illustrate underlying assumptions and core beliefs. The downward arrow technique can be used to help clients identify their core beliefs, and members can provide examples to show how core beliefs operate in their lives. Chapter 7 of the clinician's guide and Padesky (1994a) describe how to help clients identify core beliefs and the importance of describing these beliefs in the client's own words. Beliefs must be identified correctly before beginning schema change. Therefore, the homework assignment after the ninth session often includes asking group members to notice if the beliefs they identified in the session seem to be operating in their lives during the week. Clients are encouraged to change the wording of the belief if necessary to capture it accurately. They can also bring images or memories connected to the beliefs to the tenth group meeting for discussion.

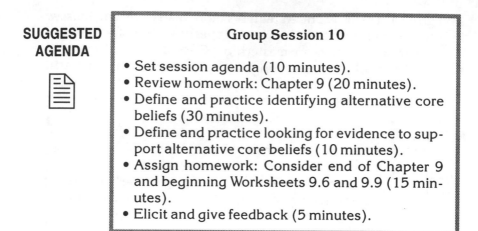

SUGGESTED
AGENDA

Group Session 10

- Set session agenda (10 minutes).
- Review homework: Chapter 9 (20 minutes).
- Define and practice identifying alternative core beliefs (30 minutes).
- Define and practice looking for evidence to support alternative core beliefs (10 minutes).
- Assign homework: Consider end of Chapter 9 and beginning Worksheets 9.6 and 9.9 (15 minutes).
- Elicit and give feedback (5 minutes).

Group Session 10

The tenth session is designed to show how alternative core beliefs can be identified, developed, and strengthened. Again, the leader can refer to Chapter 7 of this clinician's guide and to Padesky (1994a) for an overview of how to construct and strengthen alternative core beliefs. It is important to state an alternative belief in words that are meaningful to the client, even if the alternative belief is not a linguistic opposite of a negative core belief. For example, if the negative core belief is "I'm no good," alternative core beliefs can range from "I'm good" to "I'm acceptable to others" to "I'm my own person" to "My opinions count."

The process of strengthening an alternative core belief usually requires months of practice, so group members are told that they will start the worksheets introduced in the second half of Chapter 9 of *Mind Over Mood* in the group but will continue them long after the group has ended. The Core Belief Record (Worksheet 9.6) is central to strengthening new core beliefs. It is designed to help a client actively look for data that support the new, alternative core belief. Although in the early weeks most clients have difficulty seeing evidence that supports their new core beliefs, eventually clients will add to this log on a daily basis.

Group members can help each other recognize data and categories of data that are relevant and can be written down on Worksheet 9.6. Clients who discount a relevant item of data are encouraged to write it down anyway and rate its believability. That is, a client might write, "A group member told me she liked me;

10%" to indicate a piece of evidence that is relevant to the new schema "I'm likable" but that she only partially believes.

The historical test of a core belief (Worksheet 9.9) is similar to Worksheet 9.6 except that it records past data rather than present data. This worksheet helps clients begin to reframe their life history in light of newly developing alternative schemas. If clients have years for which they have no memories, they can be encouraged to complete Worksheet 9.9 for those years for which they have memories. Even clients who have had particularly harsh lives usually can find some small bits of evidence for all age periods that support a new, more adaptive schema. Finding historical as well as present evidence helps the new schema gain strength.

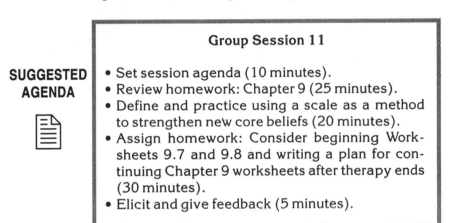

SUGGESTED AGENDA

Group Session 11

- Set session agenda (10 minutes).
- Review homework: Chapter 9 (25 minutes).
- Define and practice using a scale as a method to strengthen new core beliefs (20 minutes).
- Assign homework: Consider beginning Worksheets 9.7 and 9.8 and writing a plan for continuing Chapter 9 worksheets after therapy ends (30 minutes).
- Elicit and give feedback (5 minutes).

Group Session 11

The eleventh session continues to help group members identify and strengthen new core beliefs. In addition to searching out data that support the new schema, methods of using a scale are introduced that begin to counter the dichotomous view of experience that schemas portray. Worksheet 9.7 can be used to track growing confidence in a new schema. Often the new schema has close to 0% credibility to clients for a number of weeks. As evidence is collected on Worksheets 9.6 and 9.9, client confidence in the new core belief begins to increase.

Most clients believe the new core belief as much as 40 to 60% after several months of data collection. At this point, it has become easier for clients to regularly perceive evidence that supports the new core belief. Until that point, clients need encouragement to keep looking for data to record on Worksheet 9.6. Therefore, the final group sessions should emphasize the importance of continued work in Chapter 9 of *Mind Over Mood* even after the group has ended. Behavioral experiments are often assigned to individual members to help provide data to record. For example, the group could help a client with the negative core belief "Others can't be trusted" to devise a series of small experiments to actively test this belief. Any positive outcomes of these experiments can be recorded on Worksheet 9.6 to support the alternative belief "Others can be trusted."

Confidence in the validity of alternative core beliefs continues to grow until alternative core beliefs are just as strong as the original negative core beliefs. This is the ideal outcome of schema change work: Clients have fully developed opposing schemas, so they can perceive negative and positive data equally and make flexible choices regarding beliefs and behaviors in diverse circumstances (Padesky, 1994a). A client who believes "Others can be trusted" as well as "Others can't be trusted" is in a better position to trust or not trust depending on person and circumstance.

Worksheet 9.8 helps clients by asking them to rate experiences on a scale, rather than in the all-or-nothing terms suggested by core beliefs. Ratings can be made for core beliefs about the self ("I am strong"), others ("Others can be trusted"), the world ("Good is as strong as evil"), or for underlying assumptions ("If I keep trying, I'll succeed"). It is usually more helpful to rate the positive form of a belief on a continuum. For example, most clients experience a greater boost in self-confidence after rating themselves 10% strong rather than 90% weak.

Scale ratings are another key to the development of alternative core beliefs. Whereas positive data records overcome a client's tendency to perceive only data that fit a negative core belief, a scale begins to weaken the dichotomous view supported by absolute core beliefs. Frequent use of a scale helps clients begin to evaluate experiences in a more balanced fashion. The more balanced view helps support the alternative core belief by demonstrating that the negative core belief does not capture whole experiences. A client who sees herself as weak, uses Worksheet 9.8 to rate her strength in various situations. The ratings help her discover that she is not totally weak and that she has strength, even if it is only partially present in life situations.

The final task of the eleventh session is to encourage group members to construct individualized plans for continuing to examine and strengthen alternative core beliefs after therapy ends. Individual plans often include scheduling a regular time during the week to continue work in the treatment manual, drafting relapse prevention plans that describe steps to follow if mood worsens, and drawing up plans for continued behavioral experiments and written exercises.

SUGGESTED AGENDA

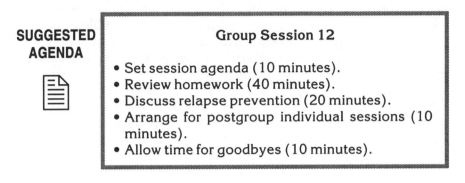

Group Session 12

- Set session agenda (10 minutes).
- Review homework (40 minutes).
- Discuss relapse prevention (20 minutes).
- Arrange for postgroup individual sessions (10 minutes).
- Allow time for goodbyes (10 minutes).

Group Session 12

The final session reviews individual plans for continued work toward goals and relapse prevention. In addition, participants say goodbye to each other and arrange individual postgroup sessions.

SUGGESTED AGENDA

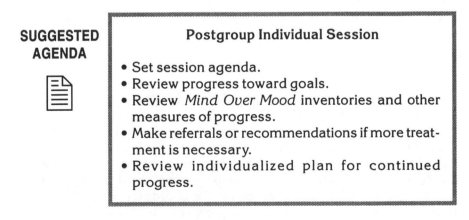

Postgroup Individual Session

- Set session agenda.
- Review progress toward goals.
- Review *Mind Over Mood* inventories and other measures of progress.
- Make referrals or recommendations if more treatment is necessary.
- Review individualized plan for continued progress.

Postgroup Individual Session

If possible, it is ideal to have a postgroup individual session to review each client's progress toward therapy goals. This session reviews what clients have learned in the group sessions and allows therapist and client to discuss alternative resources for helping the client achieve or maintain progress toward goals. Finally, relapse prevention strategies can be addressed in more detail in this session.

♦ ♦

The eight- and twelve-session group therapies outlined in this chapter focus on cognitive skill building. Other group protocols may be organized to help clients with a particular problem or to provide an inexpensive aftercare program for clients who have already completed an individual or group program but need more structured help. Group plans can be altered to adjust to different settings, parameters, and client populations. If fewer than eight sessions are planned, or if the group develops skills at a slower pace, the therapist needs to decide what skills will be most beneficial to the client group and focus on those in the time available. Flexibility is required; no two groups are alike. Client feedback is the key to proper pacing and speed.

TROUBLESHOOTING GUIDE

Different Rates of Client Progress and Skill Development

Inevitably group members learn and progress at different speeds, and it is important to anticipate differences and have a plan to address them. A skilled group therapist balances the needs of group members who are ready to learn new and more complex skills with the needs of group members who have not yet mastered more basic skills.

One strategy for accommodating different paces of client learning is to continue to emphasize the earlier skills when working on later skills. For example, more advanced group members may be ready to look for evidence that does or does not support their hot thoughts while less advanced group members need continued work on identifying hot thoughts. The group therapist can draw the first five columns of a Thought Record on the board. Using examples from group members, the therapist can work with the evidence columns (columns 4 and 5) while continuing to emphasize the skills and processes involved in identifying automatic thoughts and hot thoughts (column 3). Time spent on column 3 provides review and practice for more advanced clients and another opportunity to learn the skill for less advanced clients. At the same time, work on the evidence columns is new material for the entire group. Thus, more advanced group members begin to learn a new, more complex skill and less advanced group members continue practice of current skills and look ahead to the next step.

A second strategy for addressing varying levels of progress is to individualize homework assignments based on each client's level of skill development. This will insure that every group member practices appropriate skills between sessions. Although this chapter of the guide suggests generic homework assignments between sessions, they can and should be collaboratively set with each group member during each session. Often several participants will have the same or similar homework assignments. Collaboratively setting separate homework assignments takes extra time, but it ensures that each group member is working on a skill appropriate to progress.

A third strategy for addressing varying rates of progress and skill development is to pair a more advanced group member with a less advanced group member. The pairs can work together on exercises in sessions and/or can meet outside sessions for additional work. Ideally, the less advanced group member gets additional help while the more advanced group member learns the material more thoroughly via teaching. Not all groups are conducive to this method; the group therapist should be especially watchful of pairs to ensure that the interaction is positive and beneficial for both group members.

Silence of a Group Member

A nonverbal group member may or may not be problematic. It is possible to learn, practice, and integrate cognitive therapy skills and not be verbal in group sessions. One group member who exemplified this possibility was a man who, despite numerous overtures from the group therapist, did not say one word during group sessions. At the end of therapy, this patient demonstrated in an individual session that he had mastered, practiced, and assimilated the skills taught. Although he offered no comments or feedback to the group, he learned skills, altered behavior, and made significant therapeutic progress.

It is especially important to regularly check on the homework assignments of silent or quiet group members to ensure that they are developing skills and progressing toward goals. The progress of verbal group members is usually evident in what they say during sessions. Therapist feedback on homework assignments provides valuable feedback for quiet group members.

Therapists can also assess the assumptions and beliefs that accompany silence in group sessions. The assumptions and beliefs can often be tested during the sessions. For example, a quiet group member participated in the following interchange demonstrating the downward arrow technique.

THERAPIST: Rose, I appreciate your willingness to talk about your quietness thus far in the group. Today we're going to demonstrate the downward arrow technique, a way to identify deeper beliefs that maintain our mood or behavior. Rose, what do you believe it would mean about you if you talked more in the group?

ROSE: I don't know—I'm just nervous about opening up.

THERAPIST: What's the worst that could happen?

ROSE: People would laugh at me.

THERAPIST: The people here in this group?

ROSE: Yes.

THERAPIST: What would it mean to you if we laughed at you?

ROSE: I'd be humiliated. You would all know my faults.

THERAPIST: What would it mean about you if we knew your faults?

ROSE: Well, you've been talking about looking for evidence. That would be evidence that I'm defective and I'd be embarrassed to have you all know that.

THERAPIST: You believe you are defective?

ROSE: Yeah—I guess so.

At this point, the therapist went to the board and wrote the following:

If I open up in group you would laugh at me.
(What would it mean to you if we laughed at you?)

↓

You would know my faults
(What would that mean about you?)

↓

You would know that I'm defective.
(What would that mean about you?)

↓

I'm defective.

Rose was encouraged to do an experiment to test her assumption that others in the group would laugh at her if she opened up and talked. She said that even revealing this belief felt like a big risk. The group leader asked her to note how the group reacted to her revelation. Rose noted that no one laughed and several group members looked at her in a caring way. On Worksheet 8.1 of the treatment manual, Rose recorded this first experiment of revealing a belief in session, her prediction that others would laugh, and the outcome that group members did not laugh but looked caring. She agreed to conduct further experiments by speaking up in session to test her belief further. The therapist also encouraged Rose to write her core belief "I'm defective" in Chapter 9 of the manual and to work on it when she felt ready.

Assessing the beliefs and assumptions that accompany silence and other group behaviors can reveal cognitions that accompany interpersonal difficulties outside the group. Identification of these beliefs helps clients begin to address potential problem areas.

Finally, it is important to offer the quieter/silent group member opportunities to speak in group. Opportunities should be offered in a way that is not demanding, but rather encourages quieter group members to feel free to talk any time they choose.

Falling Behind or Getting Ahead of Schedule

This chapter outlines eight- and twelve-session structured *Mind Over Mood* groups. Even if you try to follow this outline, you may get behind or ahead of schedule. If you are ahead of schedule, continue to move forward at a pace that is responsive to your group. Use time left over for group practice of more complicated skills. Once group members have mastered the basic skills, they can use extra time to apply the skills to other areas in their lives. For example, a group member who has been working on depression can apply the cognitive and behavioral skills he or she has learned to other difficulties such as anxiety or problems in relationships.

More common are groups that progress more slowly than the plan outlined in this chapter. At a minimum, it is important that group members learn the skills that are described in the first six sessions. The skills of completing Thought Records and actively experimenting to evaluate beliefs and behaviors will help most group members improve their mood and begin behavior change.

Once a group begins falling behind schedule, it is important to review session time allocation. Consider whether too much time is spent on didactic material, group examples, or discussion that doesn't benefit the group as a whole. It is often worthwhile to ask the group for feedback regarding time allocation, pacing, and session structure and content. It is critical to spend enough time on each skill for most group members to master it. At the same time, make sure learning progresses from week to week.

Open Groups

This chapter describes closed groups: All group members begin and end the group at the same time. However, in some settings, open groups are the norm: Group members can enter and exit groups at any time. Guidelines for open groups are similar to those for closed groups in which group members are progressing at different speeds. A key therapist task is to balance the needs of the group members who are more experienced with the needs of the newer group members. By providing both basic and new material in each session, beneficial information is presented to all group members.

When more advanced material is presented in an open group, emphasize the basics for new group members. It is also advisable to begin each group with a review of the cognitive model and the skills involved in filling out the first three columns of the Thought Record. More advanced group members can explain introductory information as review and practice of what they have already learned. Thus, advanced group members are encouraged to demonstrate their skills to help socialize new group members to cognitive therapy. Throughout the sessions, more experienced group members are asked to explain principles, provide encapsulated summaries, and offer examples to foster learning for the entire group. New group members are encouraged to participate in group exercises at their own skill level.

As described for closed groups in which members are progressing at different speeds, a more experienced group member can be paired with a newer group member. This may be done to orient or socialize the new member to the group, or to help a new group member develop some of the more basic skills. The group therapist should monitor the progress made by pairs to ensure that both group members are experiencing positive learning.

RECOMMENDED READINGS

Freeman, A., Schrodt, G.R., Gilson, M., & Ludgate, J.W. (1993). Group cognitive therapy with inpatients. In J.H. Wright, M.E. Thase, A.T. Beck, & J.W. Ludgate (Eds.), *Cognitive therapy with inpatients: Developing a cognitive milieu* (pp. 121–153). New York: Guilford Press.

Hollon, S.D., & Evans, M. (1983). Cognitive therapy for depression in a group format. In A. Freeman (Ed.), *Cognitive therapy with couples and groups* (pp. 11–41). New York: Plenum Press.

Hollon, S.D., & Shaw, B.F. (1979). Group cognitive therapy for depressed patients. In A.T. Beck, A.J. Rush, B.F. Shaw, & G. Emery, *Cognitive therapy for depression* (pp. 328–353). New York: Guilford Press.

Using MIND OVER MOOD in Inpatient Settings

Clinicians face many challenges with psychiatrically hospitalized patients. Hospitalized patients are often experiencing serious life crises, suicidal, severely depressed or chemically dependent, and struggling with symptoms of multiple diagnoses including personality disorders. These patients often have poor social supports and dysfunctional family relationships. The challenges of treating hospitalized patients are also intensified by demands for briefer periods of hospitalization.

Despite the challenges, inpatient treatment has several advantages. First, in times of crisis, core maladaptive schema are often activated, so there is an opportunity to identify and clearly focus on core psychotherapeutic content. Second, 24-hour treatment is intensive treatment. In addition to the treatment programs offered by the hospital, inpatients usually have therapy sessions with their primary individual therapists several times a week or even daily. The high frequency of therapy sessions at a time when the patient is not distracted by his or her usual daily responsibilities often allows for a rapid acquisition and integration of skills.

The first section of this chapter presents a case example to illustrate how a clinician can use *Mind Over Mood* to structure therapy for an individual patient during a brief hospitalization. Later sections of this chapter address some of the ways a hospital's multidisciplinary team can use *Mind Over Mood* to enhance a treatment program.

INDIVIDUAL THERAPY
WITH HOSPITALIZED PATIENTS

Individual inpatient cognitive therapy generally follows the protocols provided for different diagnoses in Chapters 4 through 6 and the treatment recommendations outlined in the remaining chapters of this clinician's guide. If patients are suicidal, special attention is paid to the cognitions associated with past suicide attempts and current suicidal impulses. These cognitions are likely to involve a theme of hopelessness. Hopelessness has been shown to be the single best predictor of eventual suicide ideation (Beck, Weissman, & Kovacs, 1976; Weishaar & Beck, 1992). Hopelessness is often reflected in thoughts such as "I'll never get better," "Nothing can help me," "I've got nothing to look forward to," "I'm destined to fail," or "The only way to stop feeling this way is to kill myself." Suicide becomes a more attractive option when one believes that living is filled with unrelenting pain and distress. Hopeless thoughts are therefore a primary treatment target in therapy with suicidal patients.

Sometimes patients have thoughts related to hopelessness, such as ambivalent thoughts described by Shneidman (1985). Ambivalence refers to the simultaneous desire to live and to die, to be saved and to be left alone to die. A therapeutic focus on fostering hope develops and strengthens thoughts and desires to live while weakening thoughts and desires to die. Poor problem solving is also correlated with suicidal risk. Suicidal patients are less able to generate alternative solutions to problems, especially interpersonal difficulties (Weishaar & Beck, 1992). One advantage of cognitive therapy for these patients is that the skills it teaches can actually strengthen problem solving ability. For example, better awareness of moods and thoughts helps patients understand problems more thoroughly. Experiments and Action Plans (Chapter 8, *Mind Over Mood*) help patients construct change plans to solve their problems.

It is important to focus time and attention on the suicide attempt or suicidal thoughts if these led to admission to the hospital. By the time suicidal patients are discharged from the hospital, they need to view life crises from a noncatastrophic perspective, be more hopeful about the future, and believe that there are alternatives to suicide.

There is considerable variability in the length of time patients are hospitalized, ranging from 24 hours or less to several weeks or longer. The following case example describes the treatment of a patient who was hospitalized for nine days and attended seven individual therapy sessions. The case example outlines how *Mind Over Mood* can be used with a hospitalized suicidal patient. This therapy plan can be altered for differing lengths of stay, client diagnoses, or patient speed of skill acquisition. While therapeutic pacing depends on patient rate of learning and length of stay, the chapters in *Mind Over Mood* guide a sequence of skill building.

Jan was a 28-year-old single mother of two children, ages eight and ten. She was employed as a postal clerk. She reported symptoms consistent with major depression of four months duration. In addition, she described a twenty-year history of dysthymia. Jan also met criteria for borderline personality disorder. She had grown up with an alcoholic, abusive mother who still criticized Jan. Her father had left home when Jan was three years old, and her mother had never dated or remarried. Following a serious suicide attempt in which she swallowed a variety of pills from her medicine cabinet, Jan was hospitalized.

Day 1

In addition to a comprehensive clinical evaluation, Jan's therapist used the initial hospital interview to assess and record the thoughts, beliefs, and emotions that accompanied her suicide attempt. Since the goal of most hospitalizations is resolution of the crisis precipitating admission, the primary focus of Jan's inpatient treatment was Jan's automatic thoughts and feelings associated with her suicide attempt. The following excerpt from Jan's first hospital session demonstrates the identification of automatic thoughts associated with a suicide attempt.

Jan's Hospitalization; Day 1

- Comprehensive clinical evaluation.
- Assess cognitions associated with Jan's suicide attempt.
- Set hospitalization goals.
- Introduce *Mind Over Mood.*
- Homework: Complete *Mind Over Mood* Depression and Anxiety Inventories (Worksheets 10.1 and 11.1), Beck Hopelessness Scale (Beck, Weissman, Lester, & Trexler, 1974), read Prologue and assigned portions of Chapter 10.

T: Jan, I would like to better understand last night's suicide attempt. Right before or as you were taking the pills, what was going on?

J: Last night was the worst I've ever felt. I've never been so depressed. I was at home, alone, and I'd just got done arguing with my mother.

T: When you were feeling most depressed, what was going through your mind?

J: I was thinking what a mess my life is. My mother makes me feel worthless. I'm never going to get better. I just don't want to go on anymore. There is no use in even trying. The only way I can stop feeling so bad is to kill myself.

T: It sounds like you felt pretty desperate.

J: I did. And so I took the pills. I decided that I'd be better off dead than to keep feeling all this pain.

T: Before you took the pills, did you have any other thoughts or images?

J: I did think about my children, but I decided that they would probably be better off without me.

In this brief interchange the thoughts accompanying her suicide attempt have been articulated:

- I'm never going to get better.
- I just don't want to go on anymore.
- There is no use in even trying.
- The only way to stop feeling so bad is to kill myself.
- I'd be better off dead than to keep feeling all this pain.
- My children would probably be better off without me.

Jan's therapist wrote these thoughts down to be used in an explanation of the cognitive model.

In the first session, the therapist introduced *Mind Over Mood*. He explained to Jan that cognitive therapy is a treatment that has been helpful for many people who have been depressed and suicidal and that *Mind Over Mood* is a treatment manual based on cognitive therapy principles. The therapist explained that the treatment manual helps identify moods, thoughts and beliefs, behaviors, and life situations that contribute to problems and it teaches new skills that can help solve problems. The following chart summarizes some of the information that can be given to hospitalized patients to orient them to *Mind Over Mood*. It is often helpful to provide a written summary as well as a verbal introduction because patients are often highly distressed upon admission and may have difficulty remembering verbal explanations.

Introducing *Mind Over Mood* to the Hospitalized Patient

- Describe the manual and give a rationale for its use.
- Review Table of Contents; assure that pace is set by the patient.
- Discuss importance of homework assignments.
- Provide a written summary.
- First homework assignments to consider:
  Mind Over Mood Depression Inventory (Worksheet 10.1)
  Mind Over Mood Anxiety Inventory (Worksheet 11.1)
  Beck Hopelessness Scale (Beck, Weissman, Lester, & Trexler, 1974)
  Understanding My Problems (Worksheet 1.1)
  Read portions of Chapter 10 (or other mood chapter if more appropriate)
  Chapters 2 and 3 (if more than 24 hours between appointments)

After brief introductory remarks, review the table of contents of *Mind Over Mood* with the patient as an overview of the manual and an introduction to the skills taught. It is important to explain that patients are not expected to complete the entire manual during hospitalization. In fact, chapter reading assignments are often streamlined for inpatients to reduce reading volume and to accommodate poor concentration or memory problems experienced under times of high distress. For example, a therapist might highlight key paragraphs and boxes in a given chapter and ask the patient to read just those brief sections for discussion in therapy or to help complete worksheets.

A patient is encouraged to complete as many exercises as he or she can while using the manual. To increase homework compliance, therapist and client can begin by completing one or more exercises during the first session.

At the end of the first session, the therapist and patient collaboratively determine the first homework assignment. The nature of this assignment depends on the patient's current distress, the length of time until the next therapy session, and time available in the patient's hospital schedule. As a higher functioning patient, Jan's assignment included completing the depression and anxiety inventories and reading the Prologue and Chapter 10, "Understanding Depression," of *Mind Over Mood*. (Patients in considerable distress or severe, debilitating depression are asked to take short, very concrete steps, for example, reading one or two paragraphs and completing Worksheet 10.4, "Activity Schedule," with the help of nursing staff.) Also, because Jan was suicidal and expressed hopelessness, the therapist asked her to complete a Beck Hopelessness Scale (Beck, Weissman, Lester, & Trexler, 1974).

Patients who will not see their therapist for two or three days are assigned more segments of *Mind Over Mood* than a patient who will be seen the following day. Hospital programs that include scheduled activities from the time a patient wakes up until bedtime allow less time for independent work in a treatment manual than less scheduled programs, so, the amount of homework a hospitalized patient can complete is also contingent on the amount of time available for individualized therapy.

The first homework assignment could include completing the *Mind Over Mood* Depression Inventory, the *Mind Over Mood* Anxiety Inventory, and a Beck Hopelessness Scale (Beck, Weissman, Lester, & Trexler, 1974). These paper-and-pencil inventories provide baseline data regarding the frequency and severity of symptoms. Admission scores can be compared to subsequent scores on these instruments to measure improvement.

Jan's Hospitalization, Day 2

- Set agenda.
- Review homework.
- Record *Mind Over Mood* Depression Inventory and Anxiety Inventory scores on Worksheets 10.2 and 11.2.
- Introduce the cognitive model.
- Introduce the first three sections of a Thought Record (demonstrate with the suicidal crisis that led to the hospitalization).
- Assign homework: Chapters 1, 2, and 3; Worksheets 1.1, 2.1, 3.1.

Day 2

On the day following her admission, Jan's therapist met with her again. After a brief conversation to reestablish rapport, an agenda was set for the session. First, the therapist reviewed Jan's reactions to Chapter 10 of the treatment manual and answered questions Jan raised about medication. Next, he helped Jan record her scores on the *Mind Over Mood* Depression Inventory and the Anxiety Inventory on Worksheets 10.2 and 11.2 and used this exercise as an opportunity to briefly review the variety and frequency of symptoms she experienced.

The main goal of this session was to introduce the cognitive model and the first three columns of a Thought Record. These new concepts were tied directly to Jan's experience by using the suicidal crisis that led to her hospitalization to illustrate them. The following dialogue illustrates how the therapist introduced the Thought Record.

T: (*opening* Mind Over Mood *to pages 34–35*) Jan, in order to show how a Thought Record can help us understand your experiences, let's look at the suicide attempt you made right before you were admitted to the hospital. Who were you with at the time?

J: I was by myself. The kids were with their father.

T: And where were you?

J: I was at home. It was about four in the afternoon. I had just finished talking to my mom—we got into an argument over the phone.

T: OK. That describes all the information we need for column 1. You have just answered the questions Who? What? When? and Where? Now, right before or at the moment you took the pills, what were you feeling?

J: Well, like I told you yesterday, it was the most depressed I've ever felt.

T: That was the most depressed you've ever felt?

J: Yeah, that's when I decided that I wanted to die. I figured that I was never going to get better, so what was the use of even trying?

T: What other thoughts or images did you have at that moment?

J: Well, I was thinking what a mess my life was, and I just didn't want to go on anymore. I figured that the only way to stop feeling so bad was to kill myself.

T: When we were talking yesterday, you said that you had some thoughts about your children at that point.

J: Briefly. I decided that they would be better off without me. And I knew that I would be better off dead than to remain in this pain.

T: As you were talking, I was writing what you are telling me on a Thought Record. I summarized what you told me like this.

(Therapist and Jan review Figure 10.1.)

T: Does this accurately describe your experience?

J: That's it.

T: Do you understand what we have done here?

J: I think so.

T: Why don't you tell me in your own words?

J: Well, it looks like you've written down everything I was thinking and feeling.

T: Exactly. A Thought Record helps us take a closer look at what you are feeling and thinking and how that may contribute to your suicide attempt. This is the first step toward making the changes we talked about yesterday.

THOUGHT RECORD

1. Situation	2. Moods (Images)	3. Automatic Thoughts
Who? What? When? Where?	a. Specify b. Rate (0–100%).	a. What was going though your mind just before you started to feel this way? Any other thoughts? Images? b. Circle the hot thought.
At home alone, 4:00 p.m. I just finished arguing with Mom on the phone.	Depressed 100%	I'm never going to get better. What's the use of even trying? My life is a mess. The only way to stop feeling this way is to kill myself. My children will be better off without me. I'd be better off dead than to remain in this pain.

FIGURE 10.1. Jan's first Thought Record.

At the end of this session, Jan's therapist asked her to read designated sections of the first three chapters of *Mind Over Mood* and to complete Worksheets 1.1, 2.1, and 3.1.

Day 3

In the third day's session, Jan's therapist gave her an opportunity to practice completing the first three columns of a Thought Record, focused on examining her current suicidal impulses, separating situations, feelings, and thoughts. In addition, Jan identified feelings and thoughts associated with two problem situations in her life that contributed to her depression, telephone conversations with her mother and difficulties with a supervisor at work. Jan's therapist provided her with copies of Worksheet 5.1, "Separating Situations, Moods and Thoughts," to record her observations. To support learning this new skill, she was asked to read Chapters 4 and portions of Chapter 5 of the treatment manual and complete one or two copies of Worksheet 5.1.

Jan's Hospitalization, Day 3

- Set agenda.
- Review homework .
- Continue with the first three sections of a Thought Record (use other examples, particularly Jan's current suicidal thoughts or other concerns).
- Assign homework: Chapters 4 and 5.

Day 4

In their fourth meeting, Jan and her therapist reviewed a partially completed Worksheet 5.1 that Jan had filled out just before meeting with her therapist and immediately following a group therapy session. She showed a fairly good ability to separate and identify thoughts, feelings, and situational factors, so the therapist showed Jan how to complete the last four columns of the Thought Record using the Thought Record she had begun.

Jan's Hospitalization, Day 4

- Set agenda.
- Review homework.
- Introduce last four columns of the Thought Record.
- Assign homework: Chapters 5 and 6; *Mind Over Mood* Depression Inventory, *Mind Over Mood* Anxiety Inventory, and Beck Hopelessness Scale.

J: I just want to die. I can't believe I'm still feeling this way. I thought I was getting better.

T: Let's talk about what happened and what you are feeling.

J: Everyone in group therapy today was talking about the suicide attempts that led them to the hospital, and I just started feeling more and more depressed as the group went on.

T: When you were feeling most depressed, what were you thinking?

J: I felt most depressed right after group. I went to my room, lay on my bed, looked at the ceiling, and the tears just started—I couldn't stop them.

T: As you were lying on the bed, looking at the ceiling, what was going through your mind? What were you thinking?

J: I was thinking about my children and that they would no longer have to worry about how I'm doing. They would understand if I killed myself. They would probably be better off without me. Everyone would be better off without me. I'm just not going to get better. I don't want them to have to take care of me the rest of my life.

T: I can hear the despair in your voice. I know how painful this is for you. What might be worthwhile is to record what you just told me on a Thought Record.

J: I started to do that. I wrote the situation and my feeling but I didn't have time to write my thoughts.

T: Why don't you write them on the worksheet now? (*Waits while Jan fills in column 3.*) You have learned to do this really well. Now, what do you think are your hot thoughts?

J: Probably "I'm not going to get better" and "My kids will understand if I kill myself."

T: Which of those thoughts is most depressing?

J: Probably "I'm not going to get any better."

T: OK. Let's take a closer look at that. Where's the evidence that supports that thought?

J: I've been depressed for a very long time. Judging by the last few hours, it doesn't appear that I'm doing real well.

T: So the evidence that suggests that you are not going to get any better is that you have been depressed for a very long time and you have been very depressed and suicidal since the end of today's group. Any other evidence to support that thought?

J: Not that I can think of right now.

T: Why don't you write that evidence down in column 4. (*Waits quietly while Jan writes.*) Can you think of any evidence that does *not* support the thought that you're not going to get any better?

J: Not really.

T: Well, Chapter 6 of your manual will help you figure out how to fill in this column. Right now, let's turn to the Helpful Hints box on page 70 of the manual. It lists questions that may help you figure out evidence that does not support your hot thought. Let's use the questions as a guide. (*Waits while Jan opens to page 70.*) Do any of the questions seem particularly important right now?

J: (*Reading silently*) Maybe I've been discounting the improvements I've been making. But it's just so demoralizing to backslide like this!

T: So one piece of evidence that may not support your hot thought is that you may be discounting the improvements you've been making. You may want to write that down in column 5. (*Waits while Jan writes.*) Is there any other evidence that does not support the thought "I'm not going to get any better?"

J: Actually, before today's group session I was starting to feel better. I had a pretty good day yesterday, and for awhile I thought there might be light at the end of the tunnel.

T: That might be important to write down, too. (*Waits while Jan writes.*) Is there any other evidence that does not support this thought?

J: Well, in looking at these questions I know my children probably hope I'm going to get better.

T: What would their hope be based on?

J: I guess they would say that I've been depressed and suicidal in the past and I've always come out of it. I seem to go through long periods of time when I'm OK and then these other periods of time when I just can't seem to go on.

T: So they would point to the fact that in the past when you have been depressed and suicidal you've come out of it—you have survived and gone for long periods of time with no depression.

That seems like important information to write on the Thought Record. (*Waits while Jan writes.*) Is there any other evidence that doesn't support the thought "I'm not going to get better?"

J: Not that I can think of.

T: We're jumping ahead to what you will learn to do in Chapter 7, but let's try to complete column 6 of this Thought Record. To do this, look at all the evidence you've written in columns 4 and 5 about whether or not you are likely to get better and try to summarize it.

J: I'm not exactly sure I can do that.

T: Just give it a try.

J: Well, I guess even though I have been depressed for a very long time, I have been making some improvements that I may not be paying enough attention to. Even though I felt awful after today's group session, before it I was starting to feel better. Because I have survived a lot, maybe I can survive this.

T: Good. Write that in column 6. (*Waits while Jan writes.*) How much do you believe the statements in this column?

J: About 70–75%.

T: At this moment, as you are focused on these thoughts, how would you rate your level of depression?

J: Well, I'm not as depressed as when we started. I guess about 60%.

T: That's a good change. Let's review this Thought Record from start to finish just to make sure you understand the process.

(*Jan and the therapist review Figure 10.2.*)

For the next session, to take place on the sixth day of Jan's hospital stay, Jan's therapist recommended that she review the section of Chapter 5 on identifying hot thoughts, read Chapter 6, and see if she could use the questions in the box on page 70 to find evidence that did not support one of her hot thoughts from either a new Thought Record or one partially completed in the first few days of hospitalization. Further, Jan was to retake the *Mind Over Mood* Depression Inventory, the *Mind Over Mood* Anxiety Inventory, and the Beck Hopelessness Scale.

THOUGHT RECORD

1. Situation Who? What? When? Where?	2. Moods a. What did you feel? b. Rate each mood (0–100%).	3. Automatic Thoughts (Images) a. What was going though your mind just before you started to feel this way? Any other thoughts? Images? b. Circle the hot thought.	4. Evidence That Supports the Hot Thought	5. Evidence That Does Not Support the Hot Thought	6. Alternative/ Balanced Thoughts a. Write an alternative or balanced thought. b. Rate how much you believe in each alternative or balanced thought (0–100%).	7. Rate Moods Now Rerate moods listed in column 2 as well as any new moods (0–100%).
Immediately following group therapy on July 30. Everyone was talking about their suicide attempts	Depressed 99%	Everyone would be better off without me. If I were dead my children would no longer have to worry about how I'm doing. My kids will understand if I kill myself (I'm not going to get better.) I don't want my kids to have to take care of me the rest of my life.	I've been depressed for a very long time. I've been suicidal since the end of today's group.	I may be discounting the improvements I've been making. Before today's group I was starting to feel better. I had a pretty good day yesterday. I began to think that there might be light at the end of the tunnel. I've been depressed and suicidal before. I have always survived. I have had some periods with no depression.	Even though I have been depressed for a very long time, I guess I have been making some improvements that I may not be paying enough attention to. Before today's group session, I was starting to feel better. I'm a survivor. 70–75%	Depression 60%

FIGURE 10.2. Jan's Thought Record.

Jan's Hospitalization; Day 6

- Set agenda.
- Review homework.
- Continue emphasis on hot thoughts, data that supports and does not support hot thoughts, and construction of alternative or balanced thoughts.
- Assign homework: Chapter 7.

Day 6

Jan's therapist began the fifth hospital session with a review of the latest *Mind Over Mood* Depression and Anxiety Inventory and Beck Hopelessness Scale scores. Jan's depression score had decreased from 43 on admission to 31, her anxiety score from 12 to 9, and her Beck Hopelessness Score from 18 to 14. Her scores still suggested severe depression, mild anxiety, and high hopelessness, but the downward trend on all measures was encouraging to both Jan and her therapist. Her depression and anxiety scores were recorded on Worksheets 10.2 and 11.2.

Next, Jan and her therapist looked over the Thought Records she had begun. While reviewing her initial Thought Records, the therapist paid particular attention to the Jan's ability to identify hot thoughts and data and information that supports and does not support these thoughts. Since Jan continued to progress in her use of Thought Records, the therapist recommended that she read Chapter 7 (Alternative or Balanced Thinking), and continue filling out Thought Records when her moods intensified.

Jan's Hospitalization: Day 7

- Set agenda
- Review homework
- Continue Thought Record review; link to relapse prevention
- Develop aftercare plan with an Action Plan, (*Mind Over Mood*, Chapter 8
- Homework: *Mind Over Mood* Depression Inventory, *Mind Over Mood* Anxiety Inventory, Beck Hopelessness Scale; work on aftercare plan

---

Day 7

During the sixth session, Jan and her therapist continued work on Thought Records and discussed how her growing skills might be helpful in relapse prevention. Since Jan was preparing for discharge in a few days, they also began to prepare an aftercare plan. Worksheet 8.2, "Action Plan," was helpful for organizing this discussion. Jan's therapist asked her about her fears and concerns regarding discharge from the hospital.

T: I'm wondering what concerns you have about leaving the hospital in two days.

J: I'm not sure I'm ready yet. What if I can't make this work outside the hospital? I've done better in here, but I don't have the same demands in here that I have on the outside.

T: So you are feeling better, but you are concerned that you may not be able to continue to feel better outside the hospital.

J: Right.

T: This might be a good situation to examine on a Thought Record. Let's find a blank one in the appendix of *Mind Over Mood*. (*Waits quietly while Jan finds a blank Thought Record.*) What goes in the situation column?

J: Talking about discharge from the hospital.

T: Good. Write that in column 1. (*Waits silently while Jan completes column 1.*) And your mood?

J: Scared, nervous

T: OK, write those down in column 2. And don't forget to rate them. (*Waits while Jan completes column 2.*) Now, the thoughts you have about discharge that you already mentioned include "I'm not sure if I'm ready yet" and "I'm not sure I can make this work outside the hospital." Write those thoughts down in column 3. (*Waits while Jan writes.*) Any other thoughts or concerns you have about discharge?

J: Well, nothing has really changed in my family situation, and I'm just afraid I'm going to backslide and become suicidal again.

T: That's a serious concern, so let's write that down, too. Any other thoughts?

J: That's about it.

T: Of all the automatic thoughts you've identified, which would you say is the hot thought?

J: That I'm going to backslide and become suicidal again. (*circles it.*)

T: Good. Now let's look at column 4. Where's the evidence that supports that thought?

J: I guess there is no real hard evidence. Although I have failed to maintain improvements that I've made in the past.

T: OK, let's write that down. (*Waits while Jan writes.*) Is there any other evidence that supports the hot thought?

J: Not that I can think of now.

T: Let's look at column 5. What is the evidence that does not support the hot thought?

J: We talked about how I can cope with situations in which I'm likely to become depressed and suicidal. We also seem to have a pretty good aftercare plan worked out. I'm going to be continuing in individual therapy, and I can keep working in this book. You told me that I could call you if I needed to or even just to keep in contact, and I believe I really have made some important changes here in the hospital.

T: I think you have, too. What would you identify as the most important changes you've made here?

J: I feel better about myself. I believe it has to do with the change in my thinking.

T: Write these bits of evidence down in column 5. (*Waits while Jan completes column 5.*) Based on what you have just written in columns 4 and 5, how would you complete column 6?

J: You know, in my heart I don't feel that I'm ever going to make another suicide attempt. My kids are just too important to me. I believe that with what I've learned in here, I will never again get in a position where death looks more attractive than life.

T: And when you think that, what happens to your fear about leaving the hospital?

J: It almost disappears.

T: Let's complete the last two columns based on what you just said. (*Waits silently Jan completes Columns 6 and 7.*)

Following the completion of this Thought Record, Jan's therapist pointed out that Jan had not had the skills to complete a Thought Record before her hospitalization. Jan thought this tool would be a valuable asset in preventing her depression from worsening to the point of suicide in the coming weeks. Jan's therapist recommended that she continue to develop her aftercare plan during her final two days in the hospital. She was instructed to review her plans with a nurse or social worker prior to the final therapy session on the day of discharge.

Jan's Hospitalization; Day 9 (Discharge)

- Set agenda.
- Review homework.
- Review progress.
- Review skills learned and plans for continued practice and development.
- Review aftercare plan.
- Discuss options for Jan to return to a partial hospitalization program or aftercare group in addition to outpatient individual therapy.

Day 9

Jan's last session in the hospital focused on a review of her therapeutic accomplishments, the skills she had learned, her plans for continued use of *Mind Over Mood,* and her aftercare plan. She had already scheduled an outpatient appointment with another therapist. In addition, the therapist gave Jan literature describing the hospital's evening aftercare groups and partial hospitalization program. She promised to attend at least one aftercare group session the following week to report on her progress.

A review of Jan's responses on the symptom inventories showed that her *Mind Over Mood* Depression Inventory score had dropped to 27, her Anxiety Inventory score remained stable at 9, and her Beck Hopelessness Scale score was now only 9, a score indicating that Jan no longer experienced a high degree of hopelessness. Her depression and anxiety scores were recorded on Worksheets 10.2 and 11.2. The therapist encouraged Jan to complete a *Mind Over Mood* Depression Inventory weekly and use the scores as a signal for when she might need additional help. Jan agreed to discuss the need for partial hospitalization or group therapy with her individual therapist if her depression scores rose above 35, a score chosen because Jan had observed that her depression seemed more manageable below that level. Since this was the last session with her individual therapist in the hospital, time was spent saying goodbye and expressing appreciation to each other for therapy well done.

USING *MIND OVER MOOD* AS AN INPATIENT PROGRAM TREATMENT MANUAL

A number of hospitals currently use cognitive therapy as the primary treatment modality in their inpatient psychiatric programs. The addition of cognitive therapy to an inpatient program and antidepressant medication can improve inpatient treatment response for depression (Bowers, 1990; Miller, Norman & Keitner, 1989). Further, cognitive therapy aftercare can reduce relapse rates for depressed inpatients following hospital discharge (Thase, Bowler, & Harden, 1991). Wright, Thase, Beck, and Ludgate (1993) edited a text that provides detailed description of inpatient cognitive therapy programs and related research. *Mind Over Mood* can be used as a treatment manual by all members of a multidisciplinary treatment team.

The earliest version of *Mind Over Mood* (Greenberger & Padesky, 1990) was developed, in part, to help focus and structure treatment in psychiatric hospital programs and to improve treatment outcome for inpatients with increasingly briefer lengths of stay. Several hospitals used this version of the treatment manual in daily therapy groups with inpatients as well as in partial hospitalization and outpatient aftercare groups. Consistent use of the treatment manual by all hospital staff provided patients with a cohesive treatment package that linked skill acquisition during hospitalization, partial hospitalization, in- and outpatient therapy. Both patients and staff responded positively to the treatment manual because it taught skills that helped rapidly stabilize crises and provided a foundation for outpatient treatment after discharge.

When all members of a multidisciplinary staff team use *Mind*

Over Mood as a treatment manual, patients are provided frequent opportunities throughout the day to learn new skills and apply the skills in different settings. Practice throughout the day increases the likelihood that patients will learn cognitive therapy skills even in a brief hospitalization. Chapter 9 in the clinician's guide can guide therapists leading cognitive therapy groups in hospitals. Inpatient groups are usually open and guidelines for open groups can be found on page 214.

The following sections illustrate some of the possible ways psychiatrists, nurses, and recreational therapists might use *Mind Over Mood*.

Psychiatrists

Psychiatrists who are primary therapists for inpatients can follow the guidelines in this chapter for individual therapy. Psychiatrists also provide and monitor psychotropic medications. Psychiatrists trained in cognitive therapy find it advantageous to combine proven cognitive and behavioral interventions with biological interventions, especially when clients have beliefs and assumptions about medications that are countertherapeutic.

Five common themes in negative patient cognitions regarding medications are: (1) "personal strength and self control" ["I should be able to get better on my own"], (2) "fear of medication effects" ["I'll become addicted"], (3) "fear of others' opinions" ['I don't want my children to know'], (4) "problems with the therapeutic alliance" ["The doctor doesn't care about me; he just wants to push his pills"], (5) "misunderstanding about the illness" ["If I have a problem with my brain, this must be more serious than I thought"] (Wright, Thase, & Sensky, 1993, p. 209).

Identifying and testing these cognitions can improve medication compliance and can help integrate psychopharmacological treatment with the rest of the cognitive therapy program. The following interchange illustrates how cognitive interventions facilitate the prescription of psychoactive medications.

Psychiatrist: Joe, I noticed that when I said that you might benefit from an antidepressant medication, your facial expression changed and you got a tear in your eye. Are you aware of any thoughts or images that went through your mind at that moment?

J: I didn't think that it would ever come to a point where I needed that much help. I guess I didn't want to believe that I was that weak. I thought I could do it on my own.

P: You believe that if you take an antidepressant medication you are weak because you should be able to get better on your own without the medication?

J: That's right.

P: I wonder if there is any other way of thinking about this situation.

J: I can't see any.

P: Most of the other patients on the unit take antidepressant medications. I wonder how they view them.

J: I don't know about most of them, but I've become friends with my roommate, Saul, who started taking an antidepressant drug when he came to the hospital. He talks about it like taking an antibiotic—it's just there to help him get better faster.

P: So Saul does not see it as a sign of weakness, but rather as a tool to help him get better as quickly as possible.

J: He told me last night that for him to not take it would be like not taking an antibiotic when he got an infection.

P: I'm curious about whether you can view taking antidepressant medication in a different light. How far along are you in reading *Mind Over Mood?*

J: I just finished Chapter 5 and am about to begin Chapter 6.

P: Good. Let's look at Worksheet 6.1 and record the situation we're talking about. What would you write in the "Situation" column?

J: Let's see. I guess the situation would be you telling me that I may benefit from taking medication.

P: OK. Why don't you write that down in the situation column? (*Waits quietly while Joe writes this.*) Now, how would you describe and rate your mood at that moment?

J: Even more depressed than when we began talking. I'd say depressed at 85%

P: OK. So let's write "Depressed" and mark it at 85% in the "moods" column. And when you were feeling depressed, what were you thinking?

J: I'm weak. I should be able to get better without medication. So I'll write that in column 3.

P: Good. Chapter 6 will teach you how to gather evidence that supports or does not support your hot thoughts. As you read that chapter tonight, it may be worthwhile to look for evidence that supports or does not fully support your thought "I'm weak. I should be able to get better without medication." You might also want to read pages 161–162 in Chapter 10, which discuss antidepressant medication. And then tomorrow when we meet, we can look at what you have considered and discuss it. Do you anticipate any obstacle to completing the assignment before we get together tomorrow?

J: No.

By addressing patients' beliefs regarding medications, psychiatrists can foster collaboration in this aspect of treatment. Poor adherence to treatment recommendations is one of the primary reasons for poor psychopharmacological response (Thase & Kupfer, 1987). Cognitive therapy can enhance patient medication compliance (Cochran, 1986; Rush, 1988). Further, use of cognitive interventions by a prescribing psychiatrist integrates this aspect of treatment with other parts of the inpatient cognitive therapy program. The five-part model for understanding patient problems presented in Chapter 1 of *Mind Over Mood* can be used by a psychiatrist and other members of the treatment team to illustrate how pharmacological interventions (physical) coordinate with other treatment approaches (cognitive, behavioral, and environmental) to improve mood.

Nursing Staff

Nursing staff interact with patients more than any other members of the treatment team. Nursing staff fulfill multiple roles in a hospital and meet with patients in community meetings, for medication dispensation, to encourage patients to attend daily scheduled activities, and for individual sessions. When nurses as well as other treatment providers employ cognitive therapy, there can be a powerful synergistic treatment effect.

Patients often express their concerns first to nursing staff. These concerns include worries about upcoming family therapy sessions, physician competency, hospital privileges, safety of medication, and prognosis. Each patient question, request, or doubt offers an opportunity to use or build cognitive therapy skills.

Consider Barbara, a 37-year-old female admitted to a psychiat-

ric hospital after cutting her wrists. Her psychiatrist prescribed tranquilizers on an "as needed" basis for agitation and self-destructive
impulses, and to quell anxiety about losing control. Once Barbara
completed Chapter 7 in *Mind Over Mood*, the entire treatment team,
including Barbara and her psychiatrist, agreed that she would complete a Thought Record prior to taking any "as needed" medications. In this way, Barbara learned to use her agitation as a cue to
employ cognitive coping skills.

One evening, Barbara approached the nursing station and asked
for a tranquilizer because she had impulses to cut her wrists. The
nurse agreed to give her a tranquilizer if she still needed one after
they collaboratively completed a Thought Record. The nurse and
Barbara then went to Barbara's room, opened up *Mind Over Mood*
to Worksheet 7.2, and completed the Thought Record in Figure 10.3.

After completing the Thought Record, Barbara's impulse to cut
her wrists diminished. She and the nurse began an Action Plan to
prepare for the family meeting the next day. Barbara felt less pres-
sure when she realized that she could take steps to either remove
her brother from the family meeting or receive help in facing him.
This nursing intervention reinforced and built on what Barbara was
learning in the hospital. It also provided further evidence that she
could control and alter intense emotions and impulses without
medication or cutting her wrists.

Nurses need time and training to successfully teach skills to patients and provide cognitive interventions. If encouraged and allowed to do so, nursing staff greatly enhance and strengthen a
cognitive milieu (Padesky, 1993c).

Recreational and Occupational Therapists

In many inpatient psychiatric units, recreational and occupational
therapists lead three or more groups per week in arts, crafts, sports,
music, and other therapeutic activities. These activities are potentially therapeutic on many levels. Simply remaining active is therapeutic for most depressed or agitated patients. Activities that evoke
pleasure or mastery are especially helpful for depressed patients.

In an inpatient cognitive therapy program, recreational and occupational therapists employ cognitive therapy principles to maximize the therapeutic benefit of activities. For example, patient
predictions at the beginning of activities can be compared with actual experiences. Often depressed patients predict that they will
not enjoy, benefit from, or do well in activities but report some en-

THOUGHT RECORD

1. Situation Who? What? When? Where?	2. Moods a. What did you feel? b. Rate each mood (0–100%).	3. Automatic Thoughts (Images) a. What was going though your mind just before you started to feel this way? Any other thoughts? Images? b. Circle the hot thought.	4. Evidence That Supports the Hot Thought	5. Evidence That Does Not Support the Hot Thought	6. Alternative/ Balanced Thoughts a. Write an alternative or balanced thought. b. Rate how much you believe in each alternative or balanced thought (0–100%).	7. Rate Moods Now Rerate moods listed in column 2 as well as any new moods (0–100%).
Wednesday night, 7:45 p.m. Just got off the phone talking to my parents. They told me they were inviting my brother to come with them when they visit me tomorrow.	Anger 100% Fear 95% Abandoned 100% Alone 100%	They know I hate my brother. They know I don't want to see him. They don't care about me or my feelings. They are choosing my brother over me once again. They don't love me. This will never get better. (I can't tolerate this pain.) I need to stop this pain. Image of cutting my wrists with a razor. I need a tranquilizer.	I don't like these feelings and I wish I didn't have them. Cutting my wrists helps the pain go away. Tranquilizers help me feel calmer.	I have tolerated more pain than this in the past. Cutting my wrists or taking a tranquilizer in the past has only temporarily stopped the emotional pain. Cutting my wrists or taking a tranquilizer will not help me in the family meeting tomorrow.	Although I prefer not to deal with these feelings, I have to learn how sooner or later. 45% I might as well learn while I am in the hospital and somewhat protected. 40% Maybe I can talk to my doctor and get her to talk to my parents before the meeting. 60% I can take a tranquilizer in one hour if I haven't calmed down. 60%	Anger 100% Fear 80% Abandoned 90% Alone 70%

FIGURE 10.3. Barbara's Thought Record.

joyment, benefit, and sense of accomplishment at the end of an activity. Such experiences can be used by recreational and occupational therapists as demonstrations of negative automatic thoughts and how these thoughts can influence behavioral choices.

Frank, a 62-year-old male, was admitted to a psychiatric hospital in late October. As part of a recreational therapy group, patients carved pumpkins to decorate the hospital for Halloween. Although Frank received numerous compliments on his carving, he focused on a gouge that he had inadvertently made above the left eye of the pumpkin face. Frank was so disgusted with his mistake that he took the pumpkin to his room and wouldn't allow the recreational therapist to display it with the others. The day after the pumpkin carving, the recreational therapist sought Frank out for a brief individual session.

T: Frank, I'd like to talk with you about your reaction to the pumpkin you carved.

F: What's to talk about?

T: I know you were disappointed in the way the left eye turned out. Is that what bothered you most about the pumpkin?

F: I was more than disappointed. I ruined it with one slip of the hand. I blew it.

T: You see the pumpkin as ruined?

F: You betcha.

T: What did other people say to you about the pumpkin?

F: Oh, others seemed to like it OK, but I don't think they really saw the gouge the way I did. It really stands out for me.

T: Do you think it stands out more for you than for other people?

F: What do you mean?

T: I know that you have a tendency to be critical of yourself and that you are a perfectionist. I'm wondering if the pumpkin is really ruined or whether your self-criticism and perfectionism are exaggerating your view of it.

F: I don't know.

T: What you do know is that other people said you did a good job.

F: Yes. But I don't see it that way.

T: Is there anything about the pumpkin that you like?

F: Actually, the left eye was the last part of the carving, and up until that point, I was doing a good job. It was turning out just like I hoped. But I blew it at the end.

T: So you were pleased with it up until you did the left eye?

F: Yes.

T: Up until that point, what did you like best about it?

F: The mouth and the teeth looked quite realistic. That's the best part of the pumpkin.

T: So you liked everything except the left eye and in particular you liked the mouth and teeth.

F: You know, Sammy said that the gouge looked like a scar or stitches, which made the pumpkin look sinister. That was the effect I was trying to get. As I was looking at it in my room last night I could see what he meant.

T: So it's possible the gouge may have enhanced the effect you were aiming for.

F: It may have.

T: Frank, I was at your staffing this morning. I know you are working on Chapter 7 in *Mind Over Mood*. I would like us to summarize our conversation on a Thought Record. Let me see your copy of *Mind Over Mood*.

(*The therapist turns to Worksheet 7.2 in the Appendix, lays it open between them, and hands Frank a pencil. Together, the therapist and Frank complete the Thought Record in Figure 10.4.*)

T: Based on the evidence in columns 4 and 5, is there another way of thinking about the pumpkin and your carving?

F: Well, I guess there are a lot of things about it that I did well. Other people seemed to like it. Maybe my mistake didn't ruin it.

T: Why don't you write down in column 6 what you just said? (*Waits quietly while Frank fills in column 6.*) When you think about your pumpkin carving in that way, how disgusted are you?

F: Hardly at all. Maybe 20 or 30%.

T: Let's write "20 or 30%" in column 7. (*Waits quietly while Frank writes.*) Could you summarize what you learned here today?.

As shown in this example, recreational therapists can use cognitive therapy to increase the benefit of recreational therapy activities and contribute substantially to patient learning and therapeutic progress.

THOUGHT RECORD

1. Situation	2. Moods	3. Automatic Thoughts (Images)	4. Evidence That Supports the Hot Thought	5. Evidence That Does Not Support the Hot Thought	6. Alternative/ Balanced Thoughts	7. Rate Moods Now
Who? What? When? Where?	a. What did you feel? b. Rate each mood (0–100%).	a. What was going though your mind just before you started to feel this way? Any other thoughts? Images? b. Circle the hot thought.			a. Write an alternative or balanced thought. b. Rate how much you believe in each alternative or balanced thought (0–100%).	Rerate moods listed in column 2 as well as any new moods (0–100%).
Put gouge in pumpkin I carved in recreational therapy. Wednesday, 3:30.	Disgusted 75%	(I ruined it.) I blew it.	There is a gouge I didn't intend to leave above the left eye.	Other people told me they liked the pumpkin and the carving I did. I liked everything about the pumpkin except the left eye. I especially liked the mouth and the teeth— they looked realistic. The gouge may have looked like a scar or stitches which makes the pumpkin look sinister. That was the effect I wanted.	There are a lot of things about the pumpkin I did well. 80% Other people liked it. 70% Maybe my mistake didn't ruin it. 70%	Disgusted 20–30%

FIGURE 10.4. Frank's reactions to the pumpkins.

242

Inpatient treatment is usually designed to stabilize a crisis and is not meant as a complete course of psychotherapeutic intervention. Following discharge, most inpatients continue therapy in a partial hospitalization program, aftercare groups at the hospital or outpatient treatment. If aftercare providers are familiar with *Mind Over Mood* and encourage patient use of the manual, patients benefit from continuity and consistency in their treatment. It is often reassuring to patients if post-hospitalization treatment builds on skills learned as an inpatient. Prior to hospital discharge, the therapist or hospital staff can review with the patient what has been accomplished and what remains to be addressed in outpatient treatment. Sections of *Mind Over Mood* which have not been covered are often presented as a part of the post-hospitalization treatment plan.

TROUBLESHOOTING GUIDE

The Severely Depressed Patient

The concentration of some patients suffering from severe depression, anxiety, or interfering psychotic features is significantly impaired. Patients with significant impairment in concentration may not be able to read and understand the material in *Mind Over Mood*. With these patients, behavioral interventions can be helpful in the early phases of treatment. Helping the patient complete basic activities (e.g., grooming, attending a unit meeting, sitting in a group activity room rather than the bedroom) involves the patient in the treatment program and may provide a positive boost to mood.

Mind Over Mood can be integrated into treatment when patients are able to benefit from it. A patient on a cognitive therapy unit already will be somewhat familiar with the manual from observing other patients who are using it. Once a severely depressed patient's mood and concentration begin to improve, the manual can be introduced.

A first assignment might be to read about the connection between behaviors and moods, which will help explain the recent improvement in depression. Alternatively, the final section of Chapter 10, which discusses the link between activities and depression, may be a good starting point for these patients. The Weekly Activity Schedule (Worksheet 10.4) and questions that guide patient learning from activities (Worksheet 10.5) can be used to guide understanding of improvements in the early phase of hospitalization. The severely depressed patient can be encouraged to continue to schedule activities that are linked to improved mood.

The remainder of the treatment manual can be used when the patient's concentration improves and he or she can read, remember and benefit from the book. When severely depressed patients do read *Mind Over Mood*, the number of pages assigned per day should be matched to their abilities. For more detailed descriptions of cognitive therapy with severely and chronically depressed inpatients, see Blackburn (1989), Scott (1992), and Scott, Byers, and Turkington (1993).

Brief and Time Limited Hospitalizations

Inpatient lengths of stay have declined significantly in recent years as new treatment philosophies emphasize rapid transfer to less restrictive levels of treatment. Whether a patient is in the hospital for 24 hours or 24 days, *Mind Over Mood* can be used to establish a base from which further outpatient treatment can proceed. Even in a limited period of time, cognitive therapy can provide patients with a model for understanding their difficulties and offer hope that patients can learn skills to manage problems better.

The briefer the period of hospitalization, the more important it is to prioritize therapy goals. If the most important goal of a psychiatric hospitalization is the resolution of a suicidal crisis, then most if not all of the exercises in *Mind Over Mood* can revolve around that issue. If an attitude of hopelessness is contributing to the suicidal impulses, then the clinician and patient can target reduction of hopelessness as a primary therapy goal. Patients can be instructed to complete the worksheets in *Mind Over Mood* to address only the highest-priority therapy goals.

Even if a patient is in the hospital for only 24 hours, an inpatient program can have psychotherapeutic impact. Both clinicians and patients need to remember that inpatient treatment is only a portion of therapy; treatment will continue outside the hospital. Chapter 1 or Chapter 10 of *Mind Over Mood* can provide "revolving-door" patients with a new way of understanding their difficulties. Patients who find the treatment manual interesting can continue using it after discharge. Ideally, partial hospitalization and aftercare programs reflect the same treatment philosophy as the inpatient program. If so, psychotherapeutic changes begun in the hospital can be continued afterward. A seamless integration of inpatient and outpatient treatment can enhance patient skill acquisition and maintenance of treatment gains.

RECOMMENDED READINGS

Kingdon, D.G., & Turkington, D. (1994). *Cognitive-behavioral therapy of schizophrenia*. New York: Guilford Press.

Wright, J.H., Thase, M.E., Beck, A.T., & Ludgate, J.W. (Eds.). (1993). *Cognitive therapy witth inpatients: Developing a cognitive milieu*. New York: Guilford Press.

Using MIND OVER MOOD for Cognitive Therapy Training

Mind Over Mood and this clinician's guide offer students and therapists an introduction to the central therapeutic methods and processes of cognitive therapy. Therapists often become interested in cognitive therapy after ending formal graduate training programs. Even therapists introduced to cognitive therapy in graduate school discover that a one- or two-term course is not sufficient to master its complexities. Many therapists who use cognitive therapy learned its practice through a combination of reading and workshop attendance. Cognitive therapists who are largely self-taught can read *Mind Over Mood* as a refresher course in the fundamentals of cognitive therapy. Explanations and worksheets in the treatment manual provide a detailed view of how cognitive therapy skills can be taught to clients step by step.

Clinicians who teach or supervise cognitive therapy can use the treatment manual to illustrate cognitive therapy processes for students. For example, the questions and Helpful Hints boxes in *Mind Over Mood* provide a template for therapist questioning strategies in session. Suggestions in this clinician's guide for using *Mind Over Mood* with different client diagnoses (Chapters 4–7) provide a helpful reminder of cognitive therapy protocols accompanied by key textbook references. Troubleshooting guides throughout the guide alert the beginning therapist to possible sources of setbacks in therapy and strategies for handling them.

Many beginning cognitive therapists try to move too quickly and skip over the processes of teaching clients the fundamental skills that research studies link to better treatment outcomes and lower relapse rates (Jarrett & Nelson, 1987; Neimeyer & Feixas, 1990; Teasdale & Fennell, 1982). We have tried in the treatment manual to provide detailed explanations to teach these skills and written exercises to assess client understanding and mastery of them. It is recommended that beginning therapists use the Cognitive Therapy Skills Checklist on page 30 of this guide to periodically review what skills their clients have learned and still need to learn to maximize therapy improvement.

The best cognitive therapy outcomes are obtained by skilled therapists who closely adhere to cognitive therapy treatment protocols (DeRubeis & Feeling, 1990; Hollan, Shelton, & Davis, 1993; Thase, 1994). *Mind Over Mood* teaches principles central to most cognitive therapy treatment protocols. Both the clinician's guide and *Mind Over Mood* provide an in-depth description of cognitive therapy methods accompanied by clinical examples that capture the complexity of their application to diverse client problems.

WORKSHOPS

Many therapists receive most of their cognitive therapy training in workshops, which vary in length from a few hours to a few days. Although there are many practical advantages to receiving training in workshops, one disadvantage is that knowledge learned in a compressed format over a few hours is often difficult to remember and apply. Another disadvantage is that many of the details and nuances of practice illustrated only briefly in a workshop are forgotten after the workshop.

Just as the treatment manual helps clients put cognitive therapy principles into practice, it assists therapists in applying what they have learned in a workshop. Therapist learning can be enhanced further if the treatment manual is integrated directly into the workshop. Several suggestions follow for teachers who want to integrate *Mind Over Mood* into therapist workshops.

Broad Conceptualization; In-Depth Teaching

Clinical workshops are most useful if they include clinical demonstration and practice in addition to lecture. A workshop leader should establish clear goals for what participants will learn and consider what teaching methods will be most effective in achieving the goals. When clinical workshops are rated poorly, a common complaint from attending therapists is "The leader seemed to know his/her field, but I just didn't learn anything I can do differently when I see my clients next week." Workshops are usually given high ratings if the information taught is perceived as immediately useful in clinical practice.

Most clinical workshops include a summary of the underlying theory and research that support the clinical interventions taught. This broad conceptual overview provides a context, so therapists are more likely to appropriately apply clinical interventions learned.

The remaining workshop time is spent teaching specific clinical approaches. *Mind Over Mood* can help this portion of the workshop by providing concrete, standardized clinical illustrations for therapist discussion and practice. For example, a workshop on cognitive therapy for depression could illustrate client responses to cognitive therapy by highlighting the sections in *Mind Over Mood* pertaining to Ben and Marissa. The workshop leader could ask participants to compare Ben and Marissa in terms of depression symptoms, history, relationship with therapist, and cognitive therapy skill level as demonstrated in therapist–client dialogues and Thought Record examples (e.g., Chapter 7). Since Ben and Marissa illustrate two quite different depression patterns and responses to treatment, they provide an instructive basis for teaching therapists the nuances of cognitive therapy for depression.

Guided Discovery

Guided discovery is a key therapeutic process in cognitive therapy. It is helpful to illustrate and practice guided discovery while teaching cognitive therapy. Aaron T. Beck, M.D., commonly includes experiential exercises for therapists in his workshops. For example, rather than beginning an anxiety workshop with a dry lecture, he asks therapists to imagine an anxiety-provoking scene. Using guided discovery, he asks the workshop participants to identify key cognitions, affective and physiological responses, and behavioral urges. He then weaves audience-generated data into an elegant explanation of the cognitive theory of anxiety.

Questions in Helpful Hints boxes throughout *Mind Over Mood* can help a workshop instructor guide participant learning of guided discovery processes. Further, workshop participants can then be directed to review the Helpful Hints boxes for a summary of guided discovery methods used in the workshop which therapists will use with clients. Therefore, when an instructor models guided discovery while teaching, participant therapists can use observation of the instructor, bolstered by review of *Mind Over Mood*, to guide their practice of guided discovery principles with clients.

Participant Practice

Further guided discovery is provided when workshop participants are encouraged to practice therapy skills during the workshop through role-playing or participation in clinical demonstrations. By immediately using the methods taught, therapists learn whether it is easy or difficult to implement therapy strategies. Other participants and the workshop leader can offer feedback to therapists to improve the practice of methods learned. Mistakes made provide a further opportunity for group learning if the mistakes are discussed along with remedies. Innovative clinical methods employed in role-plays can also be discussed to advance the learning of attending therapists.

Mind Over Mood provides structured materials to guide participant practice during workshops. For example, therapists can do role-plays using the worksheets from *Mind Over Mood* to provide focus for therapist interventions. Therapists can do role-plays in pairs or in small groups. In small-group role-plays, one therapist acts as primary therapist, one as the client, and the remaining therapists serve as observer consultants. If therapists will be using *Mind Over Mood* with their clients after the workshop, role-play practice using the treatment manual facilitates therapist confidence for integrating the manual into therapy. If many pairs or groups are roleplaying simultaneously, a large-group discussion of learning and difficulties uncovered in the role-plays can maximize the value of this exercise. The workshop leader may choose to conduct one or more clinical demonstrations to clarify learning points still unclear to the group after role-play practice.

Another way for participants to practice and learn skills is to use *Mind Over Mood* worksheets during the workshop to apply cognitive therapy methods to their own beliefs and emotions. The senior author of this guide has taught several workshops in which participant therapists identified their own thoughts and emotional reactions to problematic clients or clinical situations. Using worksheets from *Mind Over Mood*, workshop participants struggled alone and in the larger group to use the therapy methods taught to evaluate beliefs, measure emotional responses, and plan behavioral experiments to resolve personal therapy dilemmas. Therapists report that this workshop format is very helpful for both learning therapy skills and deriving professional benefit from applying these methods to problems in clinical practice.

Linking Treatment Protocols to *Mind Over Mood*

Workshop leaders who believe that *Mind Over Mood* will help therapists adhere more closely to treatment protocols can illustrate in workshops how protocols are linked to the treatment manual. Chapters 3 through 7 in this guide provide brief treatment protocols for a variety of problems addressed in cognitive therapy. Workshop leaders can use these protocols as guides or develop more individualized protocols for particular populations of clients or treatment providers. Ideally, workshops offer a summary of treatment principles, clinical illustration of their application, participant practice of therapy methods, and time for questions and problem solving of "stuck" points encountered in the practice of skills.

Workshops can illustrate in more depth than either of the books the conceptualizations, therapy methods, and challenges faced in treating of particular problems or client groups. Using *Mind Over Mood* or the *Clinician's Guide to Mind Over Mood* as templates for describing treatment protocols leaves more time available in workshops to discuss advanced topics and the complexities of treatment. Further, if attending therapists leave the workshop with manuals illustrating written protocols, it will be easier for them to follow the protocols presented.

CLASSES AND INTENSIVE
TRAINING PROGRAMS

Unlike workshops, classes and intensive training programs allow participants to learn and apply cognitive therapy skills over a number of weeks or months, usually with ongoing instructor or supervisor feedback on therapy skill acquisition. All the principles described for workshops apply as well to intensive training programs, but students can be offered greater depth of teaching.

Personal Use of Cognitive Therapy
to Facilitate Learning

One of the best ways to learn cognitive therapy is to practice the clinical methods on one's own beliefs and moods. Therapists in intensive training programs can apply cognitive therapy to their own lives in addition to improving their therapeutic skills with clients. Students of cognitive therapy can be asked to use *Mind Over Mood* themselves as part of a training program, completing all the worksheets for personally relevant situations. Personal assignments help therapists learn what it is like to self-administer cognitive therapy during times of emotional arousal. Also, personal use of *Mind Over Mood* increases therapist familiarity with the information in the manual. As mentioned in Chapters 1 and 2 of this guide, degree of familiarity with *Mind Over Mood* in part determines how well a therapist chooses and tailors client assignments in the manual.

Many therapists struggle with the structure or other aspects of cognitive therapy. They may hold beliefs such as, "Structure interferes with client experience of emotions," "Structure inhibits a good therapy relationship," or "Structure is controlling on the part of the therapist." It is important to test therapist beliefs that interfere with cognitive therapy practice. This is especially true for beliefs about therapy structure, because cognitive therapy's structure has been linked to better treatment outcome (Shaw, 1988).

Client examples in *Mind Over Mood* can be used as initial data to examine negative beliefs about structure. For example, does the structure of the therapy inhibit Marissa from experiencing her emotions in Chapter 7? In what way is the therapist controlling in the dialogues in the manual? In what ways does the structure put the client more in control? Do students find examples in *Mind Over Mood* in which structure inhibits a good therapy relationship? Examples in which structure enhances the therapy relationship? As these questions imply, therapist beliefs can be tested on Thought Records using the methods described in *Mind Over Mood*. In addition to completing Thought Records, therapists can conduct behavioral experiments and actively seek feedback from clients regarding the impact of changes in therapist style or procedure.

Component Skills Practice

Mind Over Mood and this guide provide in-depth illustrations of the guided discovery methods used in cognitive therapy to teach clients fundamental skills for identifying and evaluating thoughts, feelings, behaviors, physiological responses, and the events in their lives. Therapists can model their own explanations and practice of cognitive therapy principles on the examples provided in *Mind Over Mood*.

Learning is often facilitated if therapists focus on the practice of a few component skills at a time. For example, beginning therapists might practice agenda setting with a few clients or methods for helping clients identify automatic thoughts. By practicing a component of the therapy with a number of clients, a therapist can learn how to vary clinical methods for client diagnosis, personality style, cultural background, and learning style. Results of practice with component skills can be discussed in class so that members benefit from the experience and insight of all the therapists in training. The group can problem solve roadblocks that individual therapists found insurmountable. In this way, therapists learn how to creatively vary standard clinical methods to provide effective help for a broad range of clients.

Case Conceptualization and Treatment Planning

Intensive training classes can help therapists become more adept at formulating case conceptualizations and linking them to treatment plans. While this therapist guide offers treatment protocols for a variety of presenting problems, most clients experience several interlocking difficulties. A number of cognitive therapy texts offer guidance and/or examples of how to conceptualize complex cases (e.g., Beck et.al, 1990; Persons, 1989; Scott, Williams, & Beck, 1989). However, it takes considerable practice for therapists to learn to develop useful conceptualizations for their own cases.

For clients, Chapter 1 of *Mind Over Mood* describes a simple approach to understanding problems and seeing connections between them. A case conceptualization should be developed collaboratively with the client, so early worksheets in *Mind Over Mood* (such as Worksheet 1.1, "Understanding My Problems") provide a starting point for problem conceptualization. A complete cognitive conceptualization of problems includes detailed understanding of the five areas of a client's life outlined on the worksheet: thoughts (automatic thoughts, underlying assumptions, and schemas), life experiences (developmental history as well as current relationships, work, and interests), behaviors (skills and deficits), emotions (types, frequency, duration, intensity), and biological information (general health and nutrition, genetic vulnerabilities, physiological symptoms, history of response to medications and other chemical substances). A conceptualization connects these aspects of a client's life and weaves a meaningful story that helps elucidate current problems and their potential solutions.

Once client and therapist derive a conceptualization that makes sense, *Mind Over Mood* and this guide provide the building blocks necessary to devise a treatment plan. An ideal treatment plan solves or reframes client problems, ameliorates distress, and teaches the client principles for preventing relapse and/or solving future problems.

Different treatment plans are followed depending on the conceptualization, planned length of treatment, and an assessment of client skills, knowledge, and options. For example, a client reporting relationship distress can conceptualize his or her problem in a number of ways. If therapist and client decide that the client's partner is overly critical and the client overly sensitive, they will probably choose to schedule conjoint sessions with the partner. *Mind Over Mood* may be used with both members of the couple to help identify emotions, automatic thoughts, and underlying assumptions that lead to conflict, hurt, or disappointment. Both partners can conduct behavioral experiments to discover if shifts in the dynamics of the relationship lead to improvements.

Suppose therapist and client conceptualize the problem instead as a poor relationship match. In this case, the treatment plan may focus on identifying the client's thoughts and feelings about leaving the relationship. *Mind Over Mood* can be used to help the client identify and test thoughts about the relationship, what it would mean to end or stay in the relationship, and similarities or differences between this and other relationships.

Many other conceptualizations might be generated for the same client problem, but as these brief examples illustrate, clients need help understanding and exploring thoughts, emotional reactions, and behaviors regardless of the conceptualization. *Mind Over Mood* helps clients learn the fundamental processes of therapy and can therefore help therapists devise a treatment plan for almost any case conceptualization.

SUPERVISION

Supervision parallels therapy by using the processes of collaboration and guided discovery to assist the supervisee in establishing a problem list, setting goals, and using conceptualizations to understand problems encountered in therapy. *Mind Over Mood* can be used in either individual or group supervision to strengthen supervisee understanding of therapy processes and provide structured methods for analyzing supervisee roadblocks.

Collaboration and Guided Discovery

In cognitive therapy supervision, the supervisor models the processes of the therapy by asking questions of supervisees to foster curiosity and to guide conceptualization and problem solving. Supervisor and supervisee relate as colleagues in an atmosphere of respect.

The following dialogue between Karen (supervisee) and Pat (supervisor) illustrates how *Mind Over Mood* might be integrated into the process:

K: I'd like to discuss my therapy with Jack. I'm really stuck when it comes to testing his negative beliefs about other people.

P: Have you and Jack identified one or two beliefs in particular?

K: Yes. He thinks other people are critical 100% of the time.

P: What level of belief does that sound like?

K: A schema.

P: OK. Have you been using schema change methods?

K: Oh . . . I guess that's part of the problem. I've been trying to test it on a Thought Record, like an automatic thought.

P: Can you think of a different method that might work better since it's a schema?

K: Well, the continuum method seems like a better match.

P: How do you think you might use a continuum with Jack?

K: I'm not sure. I haven't used the continuum much.

P: Would you like to use part of our session today reviewing continuum work with schemas?

K: Yes. If I role-play Jack, could you show me how you would use a continuum?

P: Sure, that sounds like a good idea. And once I learn from you how Jack is likely to respond, we can shift roles and you can practice using a continuum to help him evaluate this belief.

K: Good.

P: Let's first review the main principles of using a continuum with a schema.

(*Supervisor and supervisee discuss the dichotomous nature of schemas, the importance of using questions so that data on the continuum come from the client rather than the therapist, and how to help the client consider the meaning of data that do not conform to the schema. Next, the supervisee role-plays the client and the supervisor demonstrates the use of a continuum. After discussion of the role-play, the supervisee takes the therapist role and the supervisor plays Jack. Places where the supervisee becomes stuck are problem solved and alternative interventions are practiced*).

P: Has this been helpful to you in preparing for your next session with Jack?

K: Very. I feel much clearer now on how to work with him on this belief.

P: I'm glad. I'd like to suggest that you review the continuum section of Chapter 9 of *Mind Over Mood* as a reminder of how to present the use of scales to Jack.

P: OK.

K: There's one additional aspect we haven't discussed that seems important.

K: What's that?

P: How do you think Jack's schema "Others are critical" influences his experience of you in the therapy relationship?

K: Well, I guess he'd be likely to see me as critical.

P: Do you have any evidence that this has happened so far in your therapy?

K: He does get hurt and argumentative in session. I guess since I'm pretty gentle in how I present new ideas to him, I never considered that his emotion might be a result of him seeing me as being critical.

P: One of the advantages of identifying schemas is that it helps you anticipate interpersonal issues that are likely to arise in therapy. If we predict that Jack is likely to perceive you as critical even when you do not intend to be critical, how does this modify your plan for the next session?

(Supervisor and supervisee discuss ways to ask for feedback from Jack about perceived criticism from the therapist and ways to put this information on a scale. They also discuss how Mind Over Mood *can help Karen introduce and use a scale with Jack's belief.)*

P: Would you summarize what we've discussed today?

K: If I acknowledge to Jack that the Thought Record might have been a poor choice on my part for evaluating his belief, it might defuse me as a powerful, critical other in his eyes and might help restore collaboration. Then we could look at Chapter 9 in *Mind Over Mood* together and talk about whether or not he sees this belief as a core belief. By literally looking at the book together, we'd be side by side, putting us in a collaborating, coinvestigative stance. I can be curious about how the scale might apply to his belief and let him take the lead in trying it out rather than trying so hard to be the expert. This way, he'd have more of an experience of self-discovery rather than the experience of me trying to change his ideas—which he probably interprets as critical.

P: Great! You've really constructed a cohesive conceptualization of your difficulties with Jack. Any other problems you anticipate?

K: No. This seems like a good plan.

P: We'll find out. Let me know next week what happens. If things don't go as planned, see if this conceptualization helps you understand what happens. If it doesn't, we may have to change our conceptualization in some way.

K: And if the conceptualization fits, I can discuss this with Jack at some point.

P: Certainly, that might be a good next step. We can talk more about how to do that next time, if you like.

In this supervision session Pat used guided discovery to help Karen conceptualize the difficulties she was experiencing testing a client's schema. *Mind Over Mood* facilitates supervision by providing summaries of skill-building processes for supervisee reference after supervisor meetings. In addition, Pat and Karen discussed how use of *Mind Over Mood* in therapy affects the therapy relationship and can be used to strengthen collaboration and client ownership of discovery.

Developing a Problem List and Establishing Goals

Supervisees usually have no difficulty identifying particular problems with particular clients for discussion in supervision. Supervision is even more valuable if it also focuses on broader problem patterns and goals. Examples of broader problem patterns include the following types of difficulties: maintaining structure in therapy, tolerating intense client affect, devising treatment plans for particular diagnoses, maintaining collaboration with clients with particular personality disorders, and identifying therapist schemas that interfere with therapy. Goals for supervision can include working on these issues and also establishing specific learning goals for long-term supervision. Long-term supervision goals might include learning specific cognitive conceptualizations and therapy methods, improving particular therapy skills, and improving recognition of client and therapist schemas and their impact on the therapy relationship.

Mind Over Mood can be used to help supervisees identify emotional reactions to client material and beliefs that might contribute to their own problem patterns. For example, a supervisee might be asked to complete a Thought Record regarding the difficulty of ending sessions on time with a particular client; reviewing the guidelines in Chapters 5 through 7 of *Mind Over Mood* can help a therapist identify emotional responses and beliefs that interfere with ending therapy sessions.

One therapist discovered that she held the belief "I'm inadequate" (compared with other therapists). Her automatic thoughts at the end of a session included "Other therapists would have accomplished more in this session. If we continue for just ten more minutes, my client will get her money's worth." Once these beliefs were identified and tested using the methods outlined in Chapter 6 of *Mind Over Mood*, this therapist was willing to conduct some behavioral experiments in which she ended sessions on time (*Mind Over Mood*, Chapter 8) and sought feedback from her clients regarding their evaluations of the usefulness of 50-minute sessions.

Schema-Focused Supervision

Intermediate to advanced therapists can benefit from schema-focused supervision, in which therapists identify their own schemas that maintain or exacerbate difficulties in therapy. Chapter 9 of *Mind Over Mood* describes how to identify schemas as well as a number of methods to evaluate core beliefs (see also Chapter 7 in this therapist guide and Padesky, 1994a). It is helpful to identify therapist schemas regarding self, others (e.g., clients), and the world.

Many therapists who are aware of a schema of inadequacy triggered by problematic therapy situations find that schemas regarding others or the world illuminate the situation more clearly. For example, one therapist judged himself to be inadequate whenever a managed care utilization review denied additional services for one of his clients. Using the worksheets in Chapter 9 of *Mind Over Mood* he discovered that he also had the schemas "Others are critical and demeaning", and "The world operates by capricious rules." These schemas developed from how he was treated in his family of origin. Once he recognized that his other and world schemas were interfering with his usual problem-solving skills, he began to call managed care companies to discuss service denials. His appeals demonstrated that his schemas did not always accurately describe his experience. While some rules did seem capricious and occasionally he was criticized, most company representatives respectfully listened to his appeals and sometimes granted additional services when he presented his cases more thoroughly.

NONTHERAPIST USE OF *MIND OVER MOOD*

Many nontherapist professionals can use *Mind Over Mood* to enhance their work. For example, physicians can recommend *Mind Over Mood* to patients taking psychotropic medications. Employee assistance counselors may not be allowed to offer therapy to employees and yet may recognize clear indicators of depression, anxiety, or other problems addressed by *Mind Over Mood*. Ministers, priests, and rabbis often are called on to help people with more serious problems than their training prepares them to handle. Self-help group leaders may find the structure of the treatment manual helpful in organizing group discussion and learning.

Physicians and Nurses

Patients treated by a physician may not be willing or able to go to a psychotherapist. Many people who go to a primary care physician complain of fatigue, poor appetite, agitation, or other symptoms indicative of depression or anxiety once a medical condition has been ruled out. Further, many patients are depressed or anxious secondary to a medical condition. For these patients, *Mind Over Mood* enables the physician to provide more than medical treatment.

Mind Over Mood provides a step-by-step guide to treatment that can be followed by physicians and nurses even if they have not had extensive training in cognitive therapy. By recommending *Mind Over Mood* along with indicated medication, physicians can help their patients develop new coping skills that often lower the risk of relapse better than medication alone. Physicians or nurses can encourage and review patient use of the treatment manual at follow-up medical appointments following the principles offered in this clinician's guide.

Nurses are responsible for ensuring that patients follow medical treatment plans in hospitals, home care nursing programs, and outpatient treatment programs. In addition to monitoring medication compliance, nurses often counsel patients on changes in life style (e.g., nutrition, exercise) and self-care procedures. *Mind Over Mood* can help nurses identify patient emotions and beliefs that may interfere with treatment compliance. For example, many patients have interfering beliefs such as "I need to take this medication only when I'm feeling bad," "If I'm tired, I shouldn't exercise," "Since I'm probably going to die anyway, it doesn't matter if I eat properly." These types of beliefs can be identified and tested using *Mind Over Mood* worksheets.

Employee Assistance Program Counselors

Employee assistance programs (EAPS) have become an important source of assessment, treatment, and referral for millions of workers. *Mind Over Mood* can enhance the brief treatment offered by EAP professionals by providing structured therapy to supplement EAP services. Further, if an EAP counselor refers the client for longer-term therapy to a therapist who also uses *Mind Over Mood*, the treatments provided by both professionals are consistent and synergistic.

Many EAP counselors lead groups or classes that are preventive in nature or help people who do not require more intensive treatment. *Mind Over Mood* can be text or resource book for these groups following the guidelines in Chapter 9 of this therapist guide. The client treatment manual can be used to teach stress or mood management, to identify and test beliefs that lead to conflict in the workplace, or to help implement workplace changes that an EAP counselor anticipates will spark emotional reactions and challenge existing employee beliefs.

Religious Counselors

Many members of the clergy spend a large portion of their time counseling people with psychological or relationship problems. As an adjunct to spiritual advice, *Mind Over Mood* can help religious leaders address the cognitive, emotional and behavioral dimensions of human problems in a comprehensive, formalized way. People who are depressed or anxious frequently have idiosyncratic perceptions or interpretations of religious writings and teachings. In treating depression or anxiety directly, misinterpretation of religious messages often changes as well.

Self-Help Groups

Self-help or support groups can use *Mind Over Mood* to help members achieve goals. Overeaters Anonymous, Alcoholics Anonymous, Rational Recovery, S.M.A.R.T Recovery, TERRAP, and a host of other groups can use *Mind Over Mood* to help their members develop and use new tools to improve their lives. In these settings, *Mind Over Mood* can be used informally as a source for discussion and learning.

TROUBLESHOOTING GUIDE

The Reluctant Trainee

Some colleagues or students are reluctant to learn a new approach or accept guidance. Other therapists are blind or belligerent regarding problems identified by a supervisor. These circumstances tap all a supervisor's skills for developing and maintaining a collaborative relationship. In fact, maintaining a collaborative rather than critical tone in supervision is one of the best strategies a supervisor can follow under these conditions.

Supervisors are recommended to take a curious and investigative attitude with a reluctant supervisee, following the principles described in Chapter 7 of this guide regarding maintenance of collaboration under challenging therapy circumstances. If therapist emotional reactions and beliefs in problem situations are inquired about neutrally, a reluctant supervisee may be more willing to discuss difficulties. The structured worksheets of *Mind Over Mood* can help therapists identify thoughts and emotions during therapy and also during supervision.

Identifying emotions and beliefs triggered by supervision can help identify reasons for supervisee reluctance. For example, a supervisee may think he or she is too experienced to require supervision or new training. When an agency institutes a new program (e.g., cognitive therapy groups to replace former forms of group therapy), experienced therapists may resent intrusions on independence of practice. By identifying emotional and cognitive reactions to supervision or training with *Mind Over Mood*, supervisor and supervisee are in a better position to evaluate and problem solve these concerns.

Limited Supervisor Knowledge

At times, a supervisor may have only marginally more experience than a supervisee. Therapists who are new supervisors or new to cognitive therapy often feel somewhat awkward supervising others because of uncertainty about their own expertise. In these cases, we encourage the supervisor to be honest about experience limitations and form collaborative supervisory relationships that rely on mutual coinvestigation of therapy method and process based on reading, clinical trial, discussion, and occasional consultation with more experienced therapists on or off site.

The numerous primary cognitive therapy texts referred to throughout this guide should be read and digested by both supervisor and supervisee. For example, treatment of a depressed client should follow the treatment protocol detailed in Beck, Rush, Shaw, and Emery (1979), as recommended in Chapter 4; treatment of a client with panic disorder should follow the Clark (1989) protocol mentioned in Chapter 5. Treatment planning for each client will require learning by the novice supervisor and supervisee. Fortunately, most treatment models rely on teaching clients the skills highlighted in *Mind Over Mood*, so supervisor and supervisee should quickly develop a core repertoire of therapy procedures.

Novice supervisors and supervisees benefit from reviewing audio or video tapes of therapy sessions. Taped sessions can be dissected and discussed on many levels: helpfulness to the client, structure, implementation of a clear treatment plan, collaboration achieved, and focus on central client problems. Session tapes can be rated according to the Competency Checklist for Cognitive Therapists reprinted in the Appendix of Beck, Rush, Shaw and Emery (1979). This checklist summarizes the main process and content goals of a cognitive therapy session. It can be used in supervision to help both parties identify therapist strengths, weaknesses, and areas in need of additional supervisorial help.

Practitioners Working in Isolation

Some therapists do not have the benefit of regular supervision and training because their practice is geographically isolated. Other clinicians are the sole cognitive therapy practitioners in their groups or areas. Practitioners working alone often recognize a need for additional training, yet the means to obtain it seem remote. For these providers, we hope *Mind Over Mood* and this clinician's guide provide guidance. Many of the troubleshooting guides throughout both books address problems commonly encountered along with recommended remedies. *Mind Over Mood* addresses many of the common roadblocks encountered by clients along with suggestions for solving them.

Isolated practitioners also can avail themselves of supervision by phone or mail. Most of the training centers for cognitive therapy throughout the world offer long-distance telephone supervision. The senior author of this guide can be asked for training center contacts in different parts of the world. Professional books, audio tapes of workshops, and occasional travel to workshops and conferences can be used for continuing education.

In addition, self-supervision can be very valuable. Practitioners are encouraged to tape and review their own sessions. As described in the "Supervision" section this chapter, a competency checklist can be used to identify areas of practice that require continued learning. Client dialogues from relevant chapters in this guide can be used as models for therapy interventions. *Mind Over Mood* can be used with clients to emphasize development of key skills.

It is usually best to target one or two areas of improvement at a time. For example, one month a therapist may choose to improve her skill at helping clients identify automatic thoughts; another month she may choose to improve her understanding of couples treatment. Once initial goals have been met, additional goals can be set. The goal-setting chapter in this guide (Chapter 3) can help establish and prioritize goals for self-supervision.

Finally, we offer encouragement and a caution against perfectionism. Self-supervision is generally the most demanding you will ever receive. Most therapists are highly motivated to improve practice skills. It is important to be collaborative and curious with oneself in supervision. Self-supervision ideally emphasizes observation and problem solving over critique and judgment. And, of course, whenever a therapist in training becomes discouraged or impatient with progress made, the exercises in *Mind Over Mood* can be used to evaluate thoughts and modify learning plans. Just as for clients, irritants and problems experienced by the therapists can become the seeds for valuable learning.

RECOMMENDED READINGS

Padesky, C. (in press). Developing cognitive therapist competency: Teaching and supervision models. In P. Salkovskis (Ed.), *Frontiers in cognitive therapy*. New York: Guilford Press.

ADDITIONAL TRAINING RESOURCES

A catalog of audio and videotape training materials, brochures on training workshops, telephone supervision/consultation, and referrals to training programs local to your area are available from:

Center for Cognitive Therapy
1101 Dove Street, Suite 240
Newport Beach CA 92660
USA
Phone: 714/646-3390   Fax: 714/964-7312

References

Alcoholics Anonymous. (1976). *Alcoholics Anonymous: The story of how many thousands of men and women have recovered from alcoholism* (3rd ed.). New York: Alcoholics Anonymous World Services, Inc.

Allen, J.R. (1973). Psychosocial tasks of the Plains Indians of western Oklahoma. *American Journal of Orthopsychiatry, 43,* 368-375.

American Psychiatric Association. (1994). *Diagnostic and statistical manual of mental disorders* (4th ed.). Washington, DC: Author.

Arntz, A., & Dreessen, L. (1990). Do personality disorders influence the results of cognitive-behavioral therapies? *International Cognitive Therapy Newsletter, 6,* 3-6.

Barlow, D.H. (1988). *Anxiety and its disorders.* New York: Guilford Press.

Baucom, D., & Epstein, N. (1990). *Cognitive-behavioral marital therapy.* New York: Brunner/Mazel, Inc.

Beall, A.E., & Sternberg, R.J. (1993). *The psychology of gender.* New York: Guilford Press.

Beck, A.T. (1967). *Depression: Clinical, experimental, and theoretical aspects.* New York: Hoeber. (Republished as *Depression: Causes and treatment.* Philadelphia: University of Pennsylvania Press, 1972).

Beck, A.T. (1988). *Love is never enough.* New York: Harper & Row.

Beck, A.T., Emery, G., & Greenberg, R.L. (1985). *Anxiety disorders and phobias: A cognitive perspective.* New York: Basic Books.

Beck, A.T., Freeman, A., Pretzer, J., Davis, D.D., Fleming, B., Ottaviani, R.,

264

Beck, J., Simon, K., Padesky, C., Meyer, J., & Trexler, L. (1990). *Cognitive therapy of personality disorders*. New York: Guilford Press.

Beck, A.T., Rush, A.J., Shaw, B.F., & Emery, G. (1979). *Cognitive therapy of depression*. New York: Guilford Press.

Beck, A.T., Weissman, A., & Kovacs, M. (1976). Alcoholism, hopelessness and suicidal behavior. *Journal of Studies on Alcohol, 37,* 66-77.

Beck, A.T., Weissman, A., Lester, D., & Trexler, L. (1974). The measurement of pessimism: The Hopelessness Scale. *Journal of Consulting and Clinical Psychology, 42,* 861-865.

Beck, A.T., Wright, F.D., Newman, C.F., Liese, B.S. (1993). *Cognitive therapy of substance abuse*. New York: Guilford Press.

Blackburn, I. M. (1989). Severely depressed in-patients. In J. Scott, J.M.G. Williams, & A.T. Beck (Eds.). *Cognitive therapy in clinical practice: An illustrative casebook* (pp. 1-24). New York: Routledge.

Blackburn, I., Eunson, K.M., & Bishop, S. (1986). A two-year naturalistic follow-up of depressed patients treated with cognitive therapy, pharmacotherapy and a combination of both. *Journal of Affective Disorders, 10,* 67-75.

Bowers, W.A. (1990). Treatment of depressed inpatients. Cognitive therapy plus medication, relaxation plus medication, and medication alone. *British Journal of Psychiatry, 156,* 73-78.

Bradshaw, C.K. (1994). Asian and Asian-American women: Historical and political considerations in psychotherapy. In L. Comas-Diaz, & B. Greene (Eds.). *Women of color: Integrating ethnic and gender identities in psychotherapy* (pp. 72-113). New York: Guilford Press.

Butler, G., Fennell, M., Robson, P., & Gelder, M. (1991). A comparison of behavior therapy and cognitive behavior therapy in the treatment of generalized anxiety disorder. *Journal of Consulting and Clinical Psychology, 59,* 167-175.

Clark, D.M. (1989). Anxiety states: Panic and generalized anxiety. In K. Hawton, P.M. Salkovskis, J. Kirk, & D.M. Clark (Eds.). *Cognitive behaviour therapy for psychiatric problems: A practical guide* (pp. 52-96). New York: Oxford University Press.

Clark, D.M., Salkovskis, P.M., Hackmann, A., Middleton, H., Anastasiades, P., & Gelder, M. (1994). A comparison of cognitive therapy, applied relaxation and imipramine in the treatment of panic disorder. *British Journal of Psychiatry, 164,* 759-769.

Cochran, S.D. (1986). Compliance with lithium regimens in the outpatient treatment of bipolar disorder. *Journal of Compliance Health Care, 1,* 151-169.

Comas-Diaz, L. (1981). Effects of cognitive and behavioral group treatment on the depressive symptomatology of Puerto Rican women. *Journal of Consulting and Clinical Psychology, 49(5),* 627-632.

Dattilio, F., & Padesky, C. (1990). *Cognitive therapy with couples*. Sarasota, FL: Professional Resource Exchange, Inc.

Davis, D., & Padesky, C. (1989). Enhancing cognitive therapy with women. In A. Freeman, K.M. Simon, L.E. Beutler, & H. Arkowitz (Eds.). *Com-

prehensive handbook of cognitive therapy (pp. 535-557). New York: Plenum Press.

DeRubeis, R., & Feeling, M. (1990). Determinants of change in cognitive therapy of depression. *Cognitive Therapy and Research, 14,* 469-482.

DeVos, G. (1980). In D.K. Reynolds (Ed.). *The quiet therapies: Japanese pathways to personal growth.* Honolulu: University of Hawaii Press.

Dobson, K.S. (1989). A meta-analysis of the efficacy of cognitive therapy for depression. *Journal of Consulting and Clinical Psychology, 57,* 414-419.

Dreessen, L., Arntz, A., Luttels, L., & Sallaerts, S. (1994). Personality disorders do not influence the results of cognitive behavior therapies for anxiety disorders. *Comprehensive Psychiatry, 35,* 265–274.

Dreessen, L., Hoekstra, R., & Arntz, A. (1995, July). The influence of personality disorders on cognitive behavioral therapy for obsessive compulsive disorder. In C. van Velsen & L. Dreessen (Chairs), *Impact of personality disorders on cognitive-behavioural treatment of Axis I disorders.* Symposium conducted at the meeting of the World Congress of Behavioral and Cognitive Therapies, Copenhagen, Denmark.

Emanuels-Zuurveen, L., & Emmelkamp, P.M.G. (1995, July). The influence of personality disorders on the treatment outcome of depressive disorders. In C. van Velsen & L. Dreessen (Chairs), *Impact of personality disorders on cognitive-behavioural treatment of Axis I disorders.* Symposium conducted at the meeting of the World Congress of Behavioral and Cognitive Therapies, Copenhagen, Denmark.

Evans, M.D., Hollon, S.D., DeRubeis, R.J., Piasecki, J.M., Grove, W.M., & Tuason, V.B. (1992). Differential relapse following cognitive therapy and pharmacotherapy for depression. *Archives of General Psychiatry, 49,* 802-808.

Fairburn, C.G. (1985). Cognitive-behavioral treatment for bulimia. In D.M. Garner & P.E. Garfinkel (Eds.). *Handbook of psychotherapy for anorexia nervosa and bulimia* (pp. 160-191). New York: Guilford Press.

Foy, D.W. (Ed.). (1992). *Treating PTSD: Cognitive-behavioral strategies.* New York: Guilford Press.

Freeman, A., Simon, K., Beutler, L., & Arkowitz, H. (Eds.). (1989). *Comprehensive casebook of cognitive therapy.* New York: Plenum Press.

Fremouw, W.J., dePerczel, M., & Ellis, T.E. (1990). *Suicide risk: Assessment and response guidelines.* New York: Pergamon Press.

Garner, D.M., & Bemis, K.M. (1982). A cognitive-behavioral approach to anorexia nervosa. *Cognitive Therapy and Research, 6,* 123-150.

Garner, D.M., & Bemis, K.M. (1985). Cognitive therapy for anorexia nervosa. In D.M. Garner & P.E. Garfinkel (Eds.). *Handbook of psychotherapy for anorexia nervosa and bulimia* (pp. 107-146). New York: Guilford Press.

Garner, D.M., & Garfinkel, P.E. (Eds.). (1985). *Handbook of psychotherapy for anorexia nervosa and bulimia.* New York: Guilford Press.

Greenberger, D., & Padesky, C.A. (1990). *Cognitive therapy: An individualized workbook.* Unpublished workbook, Center for Cognitive Therapy, Newport Beach, CA.

Greenberger, D., & Padesky, C.A. (1995). *Mind over mood: A cognitive therapy treatment manual for clients.* New York: Guilford Press.

Greene, B. (1994). African American women. In L. Comas-Diaz & B. Greene (Eds.). *Women of color: Integrating ethnic and gender identities in psychotherapy* (pp. 10-29). New York: Guilford Press.

Hatch, M.L., & Paradis, C. (1993, October). Panic disorder with agoraphobia: A focus on group treatment with African Americans. *the Behavior Therapist, 16*(9), 240-241.

Hawton, K., Salkovskis, P.M., Kirk, J., & Clark, D.M. (Eds.). (1989). *Cognitive behaviour therapy for psychiatric problems: A practical guide*. New York: Oxford University Press.

Hollon, S.D., Shelton, R.C., & Davis, D.D. (1993). Cognitive therapy for depression: Conceptual issues and clinical efficacy. *Journal of Consulting and Clinical Psychology, 2,* 270-275.

Hollon, S.D., & Najavits, L. (1988). Review of empirical studies of cognitive therapy. In A.J. Frances & R.E. Hales (Eds.). *American Psychiatric Press Review of Psychiatry* (Vol. 7, pp. 643-666). Washington D.C.: American Psychiatric Press.

Hollon, S.D., Shelton, R.C., & Loosen, P.T. (1991). Cognitive therapy and pharmacology for depression. *Journal of Clinical Psychology, 59,* 88-99.

Iwamasu, G.Y. (1993, October). Asian Americans and cognitive behavioral therapy. *the Behavior Therapist, 16*(9), 233-235.

Jarrett, R.B., & Nelson, R.O. (1987). Mechanisms of change in cognitive therapy of depression. *Behavior Therapy, 18*(3), 227-241.

Jayakar, K. (1994). Women of the Indian subcontinent. In L. Comas-Diaz, & B. Greene (Eds.). *Women of color: Integrating ethnic and gender identities in psychotherapy* (pp. 161-181). New York: Guilford Press.

Kingdon, D.G., & Turkington, D. (1994). *Cognitive-behavioral therapy of schizophrenia*. New York: Guilford Press.

Meichenbaum, D. (1994). *A clinical handbook/practical therapist manual for assessing and treating adults with post-traumatic stress disorder (PTSD)*. Waterloo, Ontario: Institute Press.

Miller, I.W., Norman, W.H., & Keitner, G.I. (1989). Cognitive-behavioral treatment of depressed inpatients: Six- and twelve-month follow-ups. *American Journal of Psychiatry, 146,* 1274-1279.

Miranda, J., & Dwyer, E.V. (1993). Cognitive behavioral therapy for disadvantaged medical patients. *The Behavior Therapist, 16*(9), 226-228.

Mitchell, J.T. (1983). When disaster strikes: The critical incident stress debriefing process. *Journal of Emergency Medical Services, 8,* 36-39.

Neimeyer, R., & Feixas, G. (1990). The role of homework and skill acquisition in the outcome of group cognitive therapy for depression. *Behavior Therapy, 21,* 282-292.

Organista, K.C., Dwyer, E.V., & Azocar, F. (1993). Cognitive behavioral therapy with Latino outpatients. *The Behavior Therapist, 16*(9), 229-233.

Padesky, C.A. (1988). Personality disorders: Cognitive therapy into the 90's. In C. Perris & M. Eisemann (Eds.), *Cognitive psychotherapy: An update. Proceedings of the 2nd International Conference on Cognitive Psychotherapy* (pp. 115-119). Umea, Sweden: DOPUU Press.

Padesky, C.A. (1989). Attaining and maintaining positive lesbian self-identity: A cognitive therapy approach. *Women & Therapy, 8,* 145-156.

Padesky, C.A. (1993a, September). *Socratic questioning: Changing minds or guiding discovery?*. Keynote address presented at the meeting of the European Congress of Behavioural and Cognitive Therapies, London.

Padesky, C.A. (1993b). Schema as self-prejudice. *International Cognitive Therapy Newsletter, 5/6,* 16-17.

Padesky, C. A. (1993c). Staff and patient education. In J.H. Wright, M.E. Thase, A.T. Beck, & J.W. Ludgate (Eds.), *Cognitive therapy with inpatients: Developing a cognitive milieu* (pp. 393-413). New York: Guilford Press.

Padesky, C.A. (1994a). Schema change processes in cognitive therapy. *Clinical Psychology and Psychotherapy, 1*(5), 267-278.

Padesky, C.A. (Speaker). (1994b). *Posttraumatic stress disorder.* (Cassette recording). Newport Beach, CA: Center for Cognitive Therapy.

Persons, J. (1989). *Cognitive therapy in practice: A case formulation approach.* New York: W.W. Norton & Company.

Resick, P.A., & Schnicke, M.K. (1993). *Cognitive processing therapy for rape victims: A treatment manual.* Newbury Park, CA: Sage Publications.

Rush, A.J. (1988). Cognitive approaches to adherence. In A.J. Frances, & R.E. Hales (Eds.), *American Psychiatric Press review of psychiatry* (Vol. 7, pp. 627-642). Washington, DC: American Psychiatric Press.

Saigh, P.A. (Ed.). (1992). *Posttraumatic stress disorder: Behavioral assessment and treatment.* Elmsford, NY: Maxwell Press.

Salkovskis, P.M. (1988). Intrusive thoughts and obsessional disorders. In D. Glasgow & N. Eisenberg (Eds.), *Current Issues in Clinical Psychology* (Vol. 4, pp. 96-110). London: Gower.

Salkovskis, P.M. (1989). Obsessions and compulsions. In J. Scott, J.M.G. Williams, & A.T. Beck (Eds.), *Cognitive therapy in clinical practice: An illustrative casebook* (pp. 50-77). London: Routledge.

Salkovskis, P.M., & Clark, D.M. (1991). Cognitive therapy for panic attacks. *Journal of Cognitive Psychotherapy, 5,* 215-226.

Salkovskis, P.M., & Kirk, J. (1989). Obsessional disorders. In K. Hawton, P.M. Salkovskis, J. Kirk, & D.M. Clark (Eds.). *Cognitive behaviour therapy for psychiatric problems: A practical guide* (pp. 129-168). New York: Oxford University Press.

Scheidman, E. (1985). *Definition of suicide.* New York: John Wiley and Sons.

Scott, J. (1992). Chronic depression: Can cognitive therapy succeed when other treatments fail? *Behavioral Psychotherapy, 20,* 25-36.

Scott, J., Byers, S., & Turkington, D. (1993). The chronic patient. In J.H. Wright, M.E. Thase, A.T. Beck, & J.W. Ludgate (Eds.), *Cognitive therapy with inpatients: Developing a cognitive milieu* (pp. 357-390). New York: Guilford Press.

Scott, J., Williams, J.M.G., & Beck, A.T. (Eds.). (1989). *Cognitive therapy in clinical practice: An illustrative casebook.* New York: Routledge.

Shaw, B.F. (1988,February). *Cognitive theory of depression: Where are we and where are we going?* Paper presented at the meeting of Contemporary Psychological Approaches to Depression: Treatment, Research, and Theory, San Diego, CA.

Shea, M.T., Elkin, I., Imber, S.D., Sotsky, S.M., Watkins, J.T., Collins, J.F., Pilkonis, P.A., Leber, W.R., Krupnick, J., Dolan, R.T., & Parloff, M.B.

(1990). Course of depressive symptoms over follow-up. *Archives of General Psychiatry, 49,* 782-787.

Sokol, L., Beck, A.T., Greenberg, R.L., Wright, F.D., & Berchick, R.J. (1989). Cognitive therapy of panic disorder: A non-pharmacological alternative. *Journal of Nervous and Mental Disease, 177,* 711-716.

Steketee, G.S., & White, K. (1990). *When once is not enough: Help for obsessive compulsives.* Oakland, CA: New Harbinger Press.

Steketee, G.S. (1993). *Treatment of obsessive compulsive disorder.* New York: Guilford Press.

Sue, D. (1981). *Counseling the culturally different: Therapy and practice.* New York: Wiley.

Sue, S., & Zane, N. (1987). The role of culture and cultural technique in psychotherapy: A critique and reformulation. *American Psychologist, 42,* 37-45.

Teasdale, J.D., & Fennel, M.J.V. (1982). Immediate effects on depression of cognitive therapy interventions. *Cognitive Therapy and Research, 3,* 343-352.

Thase, M.E. (1994, February). After the fall: Perspectives on cognitive behavioral treatment of depression in the "post-collaborative" era. *the Behavioral Therapist, 2,* 48-51.

Thase, M.E., Bowler, K., & Harden, T. (1991). Cognitive behavior therapy of endogenous depression: Part 2: Preliminary findings in 16 unmedicated inpatients. *Behavior Therapy, 22,* 469-477.

Thase, M.E., & Kupfer, D.J. (1987). Characteristics of treatment resistant depression. In J. Zohar & R.H. Belmaker (Eds.), *Treating resistant depression* (pp. 23-45). New York: PMA Publishing.

van Velzen, C.J.M., & Emmelkamp, P.M.G. (1995, July). The influence of personality disorders on treatment outcome of social phobia. In C. van Velsen & L. Dreessen (Chairs), *Impact of personality disorders on cognitive-behavioural treatment of Axis I disorders.* Symposium conducted at the meeting of the World Congress of Behavioral and Cognitive Therapies, Copenhagen, Denmark.

Weishaar, M.E., & Beck, A.T. (1992). Hopelessness and suicide. *International Review of Psychiatry, 4,* 177-184.

Woody, G.E., McLellan, A.T., Luborsky, L., O'Brien, C.P., Blaine, J., Fox, S., Herman, I., & Beck, A.T. (1984). Severity of psychiatric symptoms as a predictor of benefits from psychotherapy: The Veterans Administration-Penn Study. *American Journal of Psychiatry, 141,* 1172-1177.

Wright, J.H., Thase, M.E., Beck, A.T., & Ludgate, J.W. (Eds.). (1993). *Cognitive therapy with inpatients: Developing a cognitive milieu.* New York: Guilford Press.

Wright, J.H., Thase, M.E., & Sensky, T. (1993). Cognitive and biological therapies: A combined approach. In J.H. Wright, M.E. Thase, A.T. Beck, & J.W. Ludgate (Eds.), *Cognitive therapy with inpatients: Developing a cognitive milieu* (pp. 193-218). New York: Guilford Press.

Wright, J.H., & Davis, D. (1994). The therapeutic relationship in cognitive-behavioral therapy: Patient perceptions and therapist responses. *Cognitive and Behavioral Practice, 1,* 25-45.

Index

Love is Never Enough (Beck), 116, 120, 264

Medication therapy, 20, 22, 28, 79, 178, 238, 259
  compliance with, 235–237
  negative patient cognitions regarding, 235–237
  reliance on, 99–102
Metaphor, use of, 38, 163–164
Middle Eastern cultures, 48
Mind Over Mood; see Client treatment manual
Moods, 17, 32, 191
  in borderline personality disorder, 134, 154
  fluctuating, 124, 166
  identifying, 109, 156, 188
  rating, 192, 201

Narcissistic personality disorder, 132, 133–134
Narcotics Anonymous, 112
Native American culture, 40
Negativity, 4, 74–75, 80, 173
Nurses, 237–238, 259

Obsessive–compulsive disorder (OCD), 28, 82, 90–92
  treatment for, 90–91, 105
Obsessive–compulsive personality disorder (OCPD), 132, 133
Outcome studies, 69–70, 83, 91, 132, 234
Overeaters Anonymous, 260

Panic attacks, 85, 103
Panic disorder, 40, 44, 69, 83–88
  with agoraphobia, 90
  treatment for, 83, 85–88, 105
Paranoid behaviors, 150
Perfectionism, 82, 103, 115, 132, 133, 158–159, 240–241
  in therapist self-supervision, 263
Personality disorders, 16–17, 121–164, 216; *see also* various personality disorders
  beliefs about change in, 157, 164

objections to treatment manual in, 156
and repetition, 135
schemas-maintaining, 123
and therapeutic relationship, 157
treatment of, 5, 123, 137–164
Phobias, 82, 88–90; *see also* Agoraphobia
  social, 88–89, 103
  treatment for, 105
Physicians, primary care, 259
Positive data log; *see* Core Belief Record
Posttraumatic stress disorder, 82, 92–93, 105, 172, 176
Psychiatrists, 235–237; *see also* Therapists

Racism, 44–45, 54–55
Rational Recovery, 112, 178, 260
Recreational therapy, 238, 240–243
Relapse prevention, 70, 112, 117, 203, 209, 234
Relationship problems, 116–119, 169, 174
  core beliefs in, 117–118
  most common feelings in, 117
Religious beliefs, 47, 50–51
  Buddhist, 47
  fundamentalist Christian, 50–51
  Hindu, 47–48
  Mormon, 51
Religious counselors, 258, 260
Repetition needs, 135
Response prevention, 91, 105
Responsibility Pies, 91, 112
Role playing, 24, 104, 153, 155, 249–250

Scale, use of, 136–137, 140–143, 144, 188, 207, 208; *see also* Continuum methods
Schemas, 5, 29, 35, 121–123, 128, 200, 204–220
  alternative, 206, 208
  and anxiety, 83
  changing, 138–140, 143, 150, 208
  and culture, 39, 40, 48, 52

THERAPIST FEEDBACK ON *MIND OVER MOOD*

Thank you for selecting *Mind Over Mood* as a treatment manual. We appreciate your feedback which helps us evaluate the strengths and weaknesses of the book.

1. What were the diagnoses for the client(s) for which you used the manual?

2. In what session did you generally begin using the manual?

3. How much time did you spend introducing and explaining the treatment manual to the client?

4. Did the client bring the manual to sessions regularly? _____Yes _____No

5. Did you asign the chapters in the order written? _____Yes _____No

COMMENTS:_____

_____

6. What was best about the treatment manual?

7. What were the shortcomings of the treatment manual?

8. Rate how useful you found the treatment manual overall?

|		|		|		|		|
Not at all Useful		Slightly Useful		Somewhat Useful		Very Useful		Extremely Useful

9. What spontaneous comments, if any, did your client(s) make to you about the manual?

Thank you for completing this form (or a photocopy). Please mail to:
Christine Padesky, Ph.D., Center for Cognitive Therapy,
1101 Dove Street, Suite #240, New Port Beach, CA 92660

(Optional)

Name: _____Degree: _____

Address:_____

State/Postal Code/Country: _____

Phone Number: _____

Mind Over Mood
A Cognitive Therapy Treatment Manual for Clients
Dennis Greenberger and Christine A. Padesky

1995, Paperback, 243 Pages, 8½" x 11" with "open-flat" binding
ISBN 0-89862-128-3, Cat. #2128, $19.95

MIND OVER MOOD Quantity Discounts

For multiple copies of *Mind Over Mood,* calculate the following discount rates against the list price to get the unit discount price. Then simply multiply the discount price times the quantity you are ordering. Add 5% of your total order for shipping.

Quantity	List Price	Discount	Price Per Book
1 book	$19.95	—	$19.95
2-12 books		20% off list price	$15.96
13-24 books		30% off list price	$13.97
25 copies or more		33% off list price	$13.37

To order, please call toll-free 1-800-365-7006 or photocopy and use the coupon below.

- -

Guilford Publications, Inc.

Dept. IV, 72 Spring Street,
New York, NY 10012

C **CALL TOLL FREE**
(800) 365-7006
FAX (212) 966-6708

Name

Institution

Address   Rm./Apt. No.

City

State   Zip

Daytime Phone No.

Guilford Account No. (if known)

☐ Please send me a copy
of your catalog, Cat. #CAT.

Qty	Cat. #	Title	Price	Amount
	2128	Mind Over Mood	*	

* See Quantity Discount Schedule above

** Shipping (via UPS):
Add $3.50 for one book, or, for multiple copy orders, add 5% of total order.

**Shipping	
Subtotal	
Sales Tax (NY and PA residents only)	
TOTAL	

METHOD OF PAYMENT

☐ Check or Money Order Enclosed
☐ Institutional P.O. Attached

BILL MY: ☐ MasterCard   ☐ VISA   ☐ AMEX

Acct. #

☐☐☐☐ ☐☐☐☐ ☐☐☐☐ ☐☐☐☐

Expiration Date
Month   Year

☐☐ ☐☐

Signature *(required on all credit card orders)*